Crochet:

Huge Collection of Afghan and Tunisian Crochet Projects in One Book

Table of Contents

Introduction

From the primitive ages, human races possessed different skills like hunting, gathering and trapping etc. humans acquired these skills for their better survival. With the passage of time, humans went through different technological developmental phases. Humans gained success in every corner of the world. One thing which is quite appreciative, humans didn't forget their norms.

Stitching and sewing was the famous activity among women in primitive times. There are evident from the history which shows that sewing was an essential component of human households. Now, stitching is practiced widely across the world. Humans wear stitched clothes to cover themselves.

Crochet!!! Have you heard this name before? May be few of you have heard of this before. May be there are some thrifty ones among you....who may know this art or skill. Crochet is a process or art of creating fabric or a pattern by interconnecting loops of yarn, thread, or fibers of other materials using a crochet hook.

The word crochet has a French origin and it is a derivative of the word *crochet* which means small hook. Hooks are made up of materials such as plastic, wood and metal etc. hooks are manufactured commercially and they are also manufactured in artisan workshops.

There are a few differences between crochet and knitting. The major difference is in the tools used for their production. Other than that stitches in crochet are usually completed before starting the next one, while knitting keeps a large number of stitches open at a time.

There are different types of stitches involved in crochet making like single crochet stitch, double crochet stitch, and half double crochet stitches. Using these different kinds of stitches, one can make many different kinds of patterns. Crochets are also differentiated on the basis of colors used in making of their patterns. Crocheting is a beautiful that will help you spend your time in some healthy activity.

Chapter 1- Essential requirements of crocheting

The first known studied patterns for crocheting were printed in 1824. The origins of crocheting are vague, yet Lis Paludan suggests that crochet emerged like traditional craft in Iran, China and South America.

Crocheting is a beautiful art or skill that is usually mastered by women. Different colours and patterns add to the beauty of this art. There are a few requirements, without which crocheting is incomplete.

The crochet Afghan will start with a slip knot and chain stitch followed by series of stitches. A slip knot is really important in the crochet. The slip knot on the crochet hook will be almost 6 inches from the free end of the yarn. You may start by creating a loop with the help of yarn and make sure to have the free end dangling behind the loop.

See the following image:

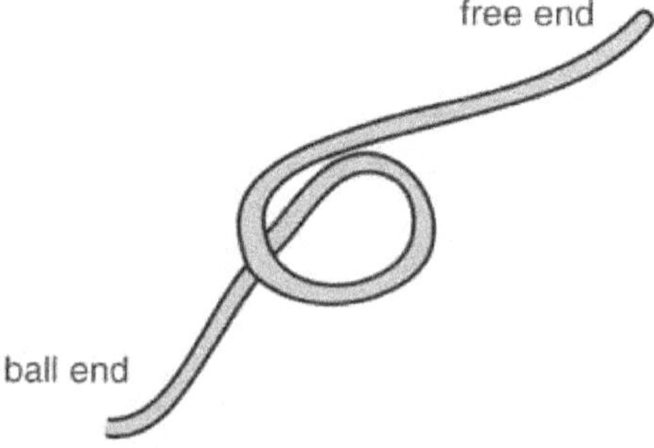

Now insert the crochet hook in the center of the loop and clasp the free end as per the below illustration.

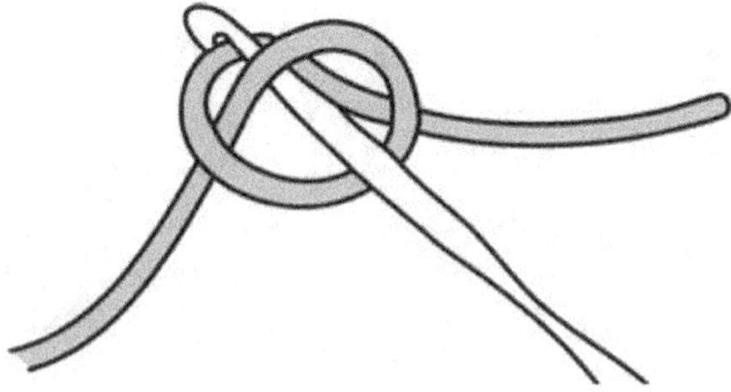

It is time to pull the yarn through and up onto the working area of the hook. See the image below:

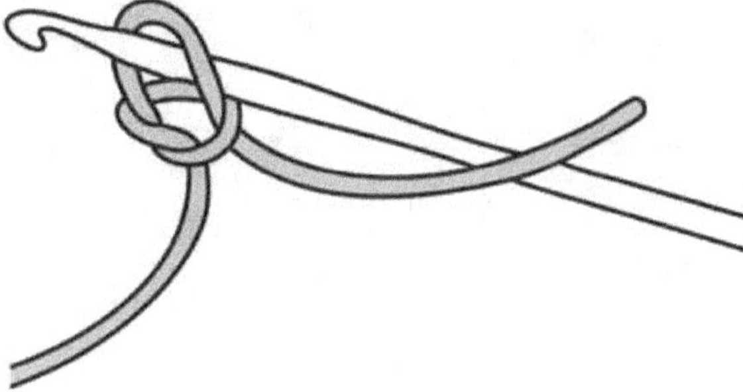

It is time to pull the free end of the yarn to make a tight loop as per the image below. The loop on the hook should be solid, but it should be loose enough to slide on the hook easily. Make sure to have almost 6-inch yarn end.

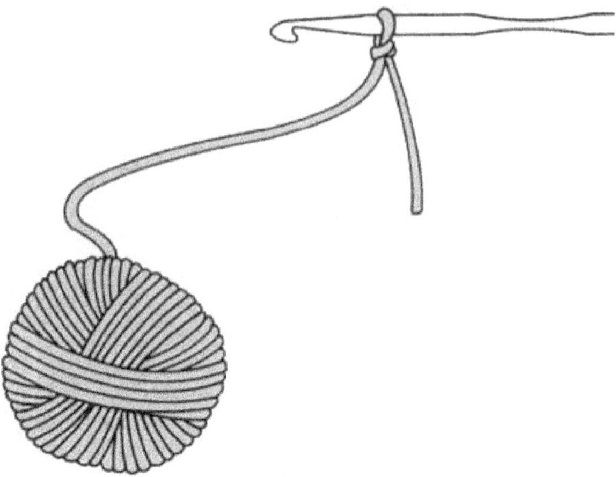

After wrapping the yarn, just hold the bottom of the slip knot using your thumb and index finger of the left hand.

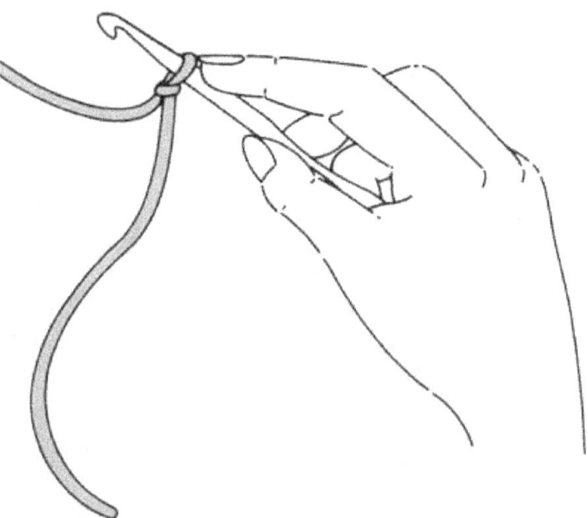

In this step, you will bring the yarn on the crochet hook from the back and hook it just like shown in the image. Pull the yarn through the ring from the rear to front and fasten it as per the image. You can make one chain stitch to start your working area.

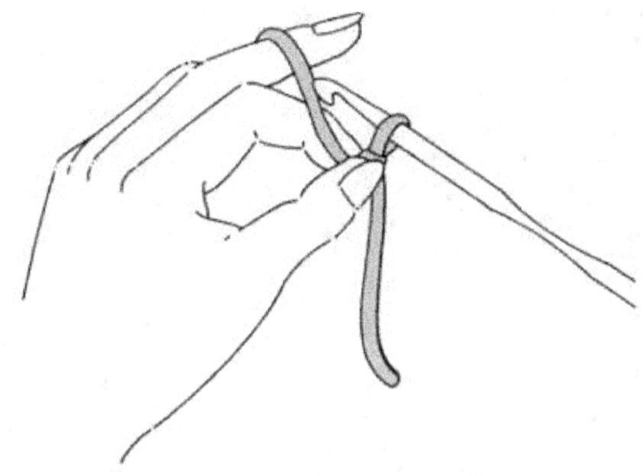

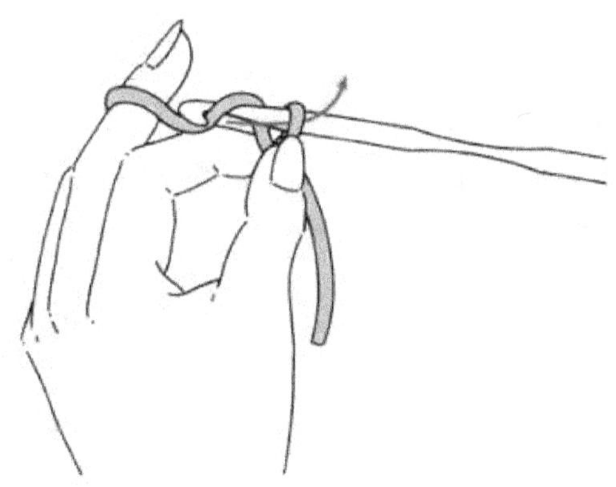

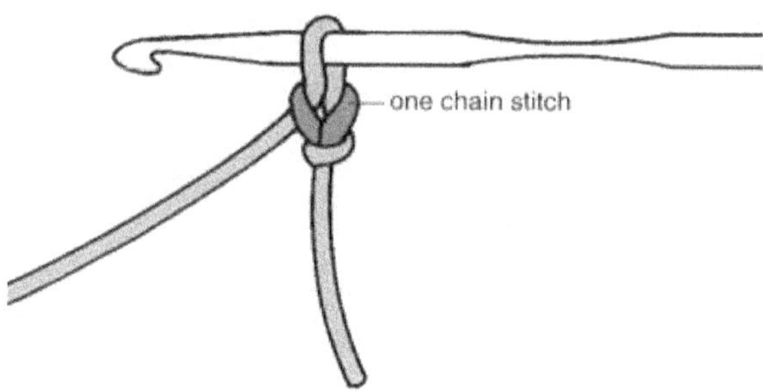

You need to control the base of the slip knot and carry the yarn on the crochet hook from back to front. Clasp it and drag throughout the loop on the fastener. It will be better to make another chain stitch and repeat an additional chain.

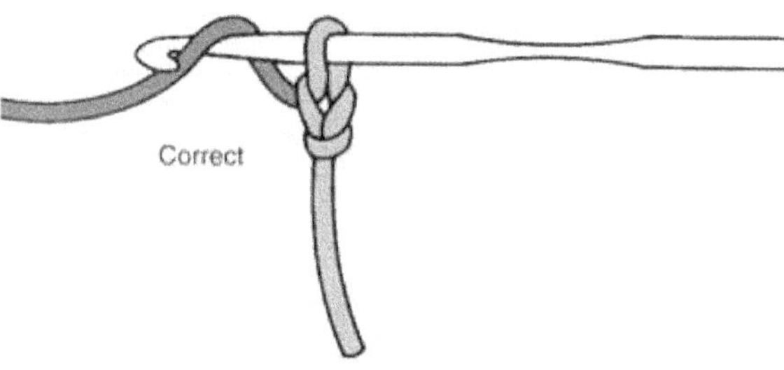

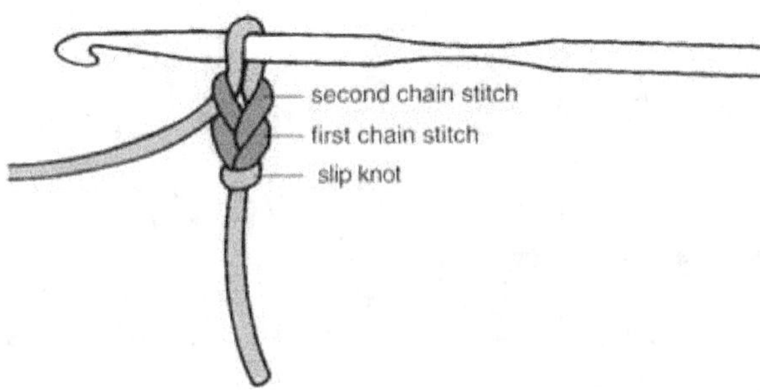

Make sure to move the left thumb and index finger on the chain close to the crochet hook after each new stitch. It will help you to control the work in a better way and pull each new stitch on the working area of the hook; or else, the initial chain stitch will be really tight.

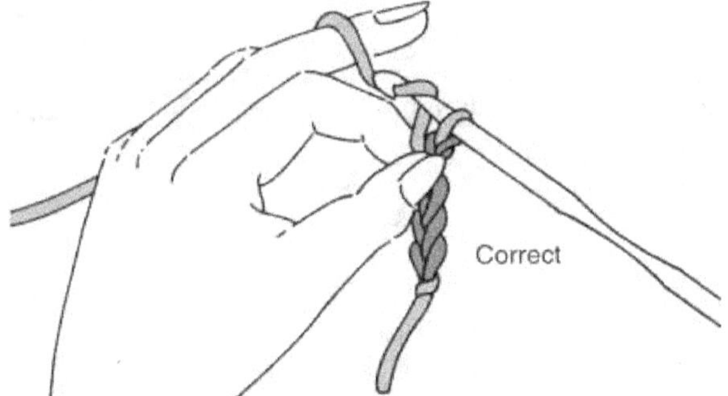

Make sure to practice chain until you become comfortable with the grip on the hook and flow of the yarn. Initially, the work may be irregular and the stitches may be loose and tight. There is no need to worry because you are in the learning phase and you will learn everything with practice. As you increase your skill level, the chains will be firm and even in sizes. While you are learning, it will be good to make loose chains.

Basic Afghan Stitch

The basic Afghan stitches are looked like little squares and these are basic whole rows of stitches on the hook that will help you to make the second row. The Afghan hooks are long and have caps or stopper to hold the stitches. These are available in a variety of sizes and lengths.

Chain almost 16 stitches for your base chain.

In the Afghan stitches, you have to pull loops through the current stitches. It is time to start a foundation row.

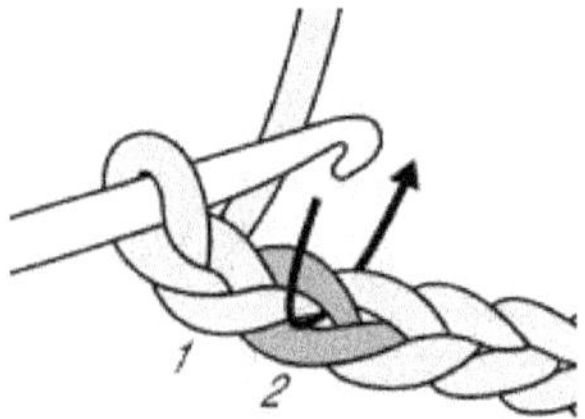

You will interleave the hook in the 2nd chain (ch) from the hook. Begin counting stitches from the stitches straight under the loop on your hook.

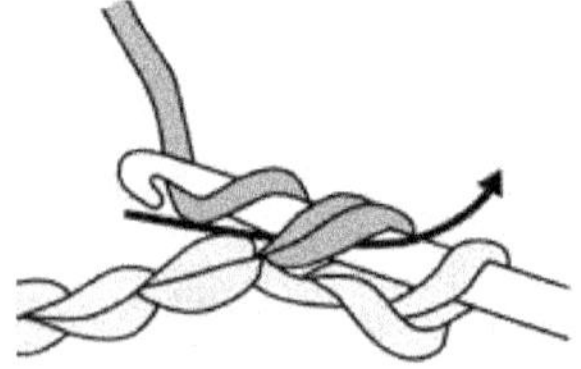

Now yarn over (YO) the fastener and drag your yarn throughout the chain stitch. There should be two loops on the fastener.

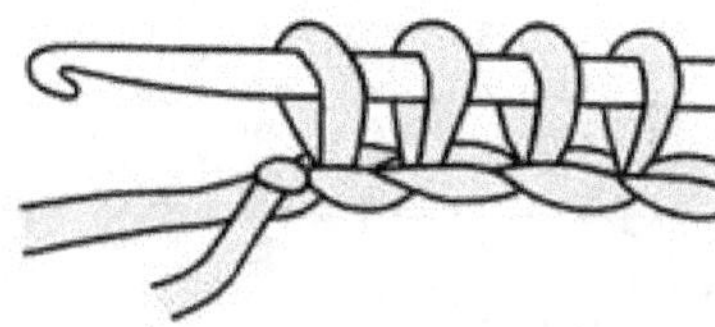

Put on your hook in the subsequent chain and replicate the earlier step in each chain transversely the base chain.

The hook will have almost 16 loops and one loop may be in the each foundation chain. This will help you to make the first half of the foundation row of Afghan stitch can complete now.

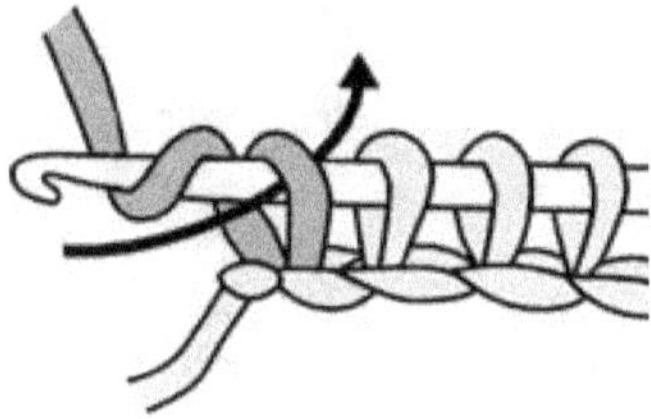

Yarn over (YO) and drag your yarn from one loop on the hook. Now work with the one loop on this step.

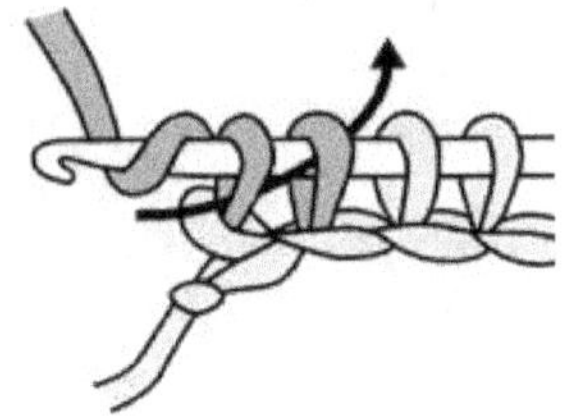

It is time to yarn over the fastener and pull your thread via the next 2 loops on the hook.

Replicate the procedure in this step crossways the row until there would be only 1 loop on the hook. Your foundation row is successfully done and there is only one loop on the hook. It would be considered as the first stitch of the subsequent row.

Now pop in the hook at the rear of the next vertical bar in the row beneath. There is no need to work on the vertical bar directly under the loop on your hook.

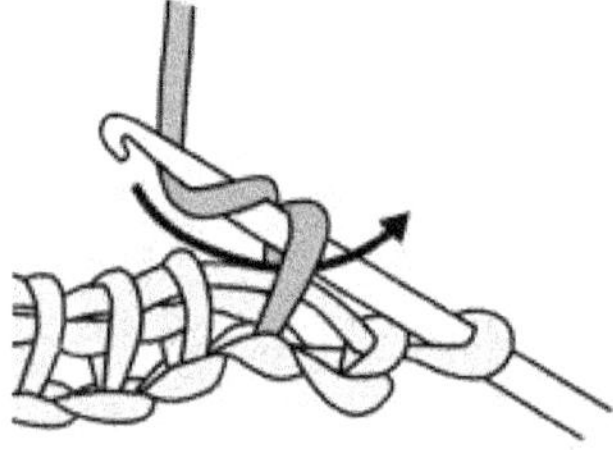

Yarn over (YO) the fastener and drag the yarn via the stitch. Replicate the previous step and this step in every vertical bar crossways the line up until you access the next-to-last stitch.

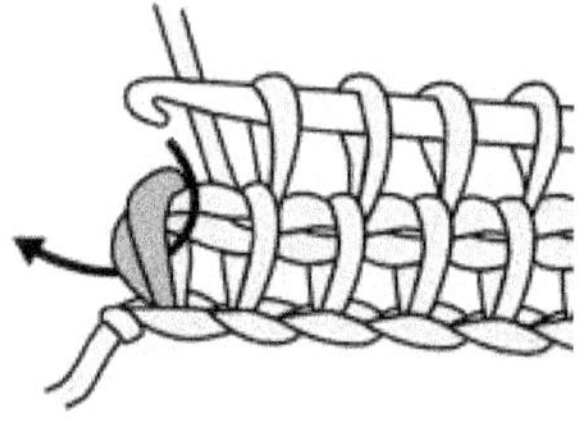

Pop in the hook under the preceding 2 vertical bars at the last part of the row. These bars will be used to finish the row.

YO the fastener and draw your yarn throughout the vertical bars.

There should be 16 loops on the hook and the initial half of the row is complete now.

Now YO the hook and drag your yarn via 1 loop on the hook. Make sure to work on one loop only.

It is time to yarn over the fastener and drag the yarn via the subsequent 2 loops on the hook. Replicate this step crossways the row until there will be only one loop on the hook. Your second row will be finished now.

You will continue your work on the rows of basic Afghan stitch until you are comfortable with the technique. You can practice a swatch of 4 inches.

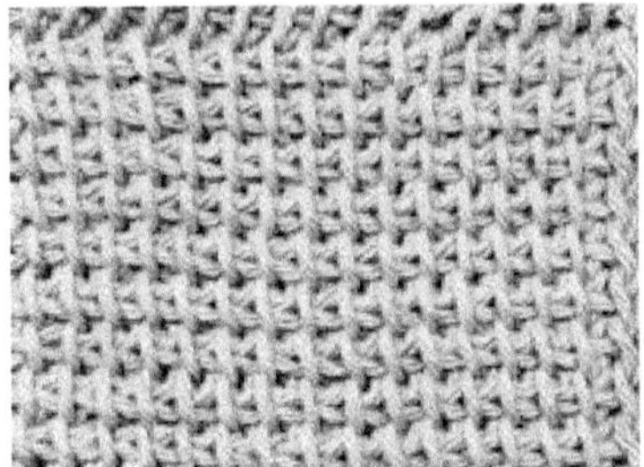

It is time to work on the slip stitch under the every vertical bar crossways the last row to end each swatch. It is important to bind off the last row because without binding, there will be a gap in the stitches.

Instructions to Make Double Crochet

The double crochet is often abbreviated as dc and it is the most common crochet stitch that is double in the length of the single crochet. It is the most common stitch and is solid for sweaters, placements, Afghans and other decoration items.

Make a Chain containing 18 chain stitches

The initial 15 chain stitches will make a foundation chain and the remaining 3 may make your turning chain.

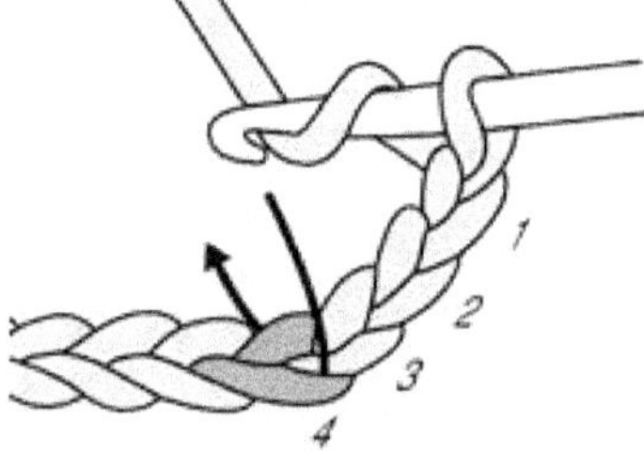

Now yarn over the hook and pop in your hook in the 2 front loops and under the rear knock loop of the 4th chain from the fastener.

You have to yarn over from rear to front.

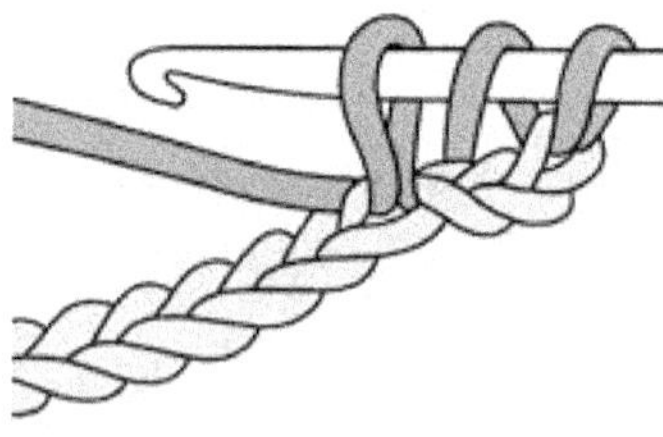

YO the fastener and softly drag the enfold fastener throughout the middle of the chain stitch, hauling the enfolding yarn throughout the stitch.

There will be 3 loops on the hook.

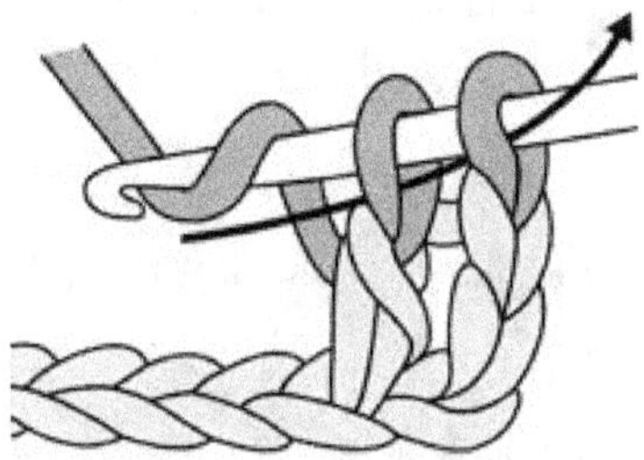

YO the fastener and drag your yarn throughout the initial 2 loops on your fastener.

In this step, you will start the dc (double crochet) stitch.

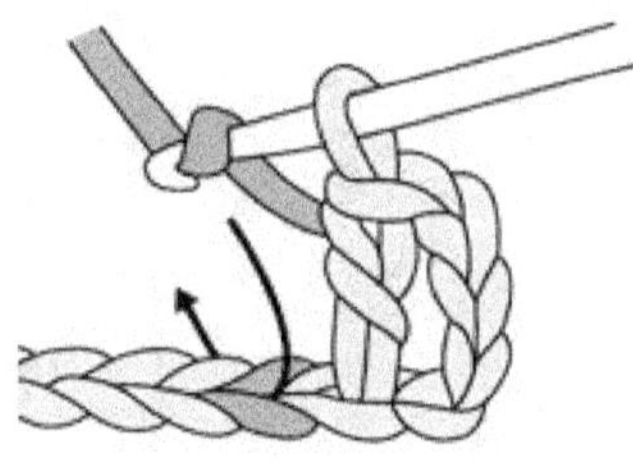

Now YO the clasp and drag your thread throughout the preceding 2 loops on the fastener.

One dc stitch is complete and there will be one loop on the hook.

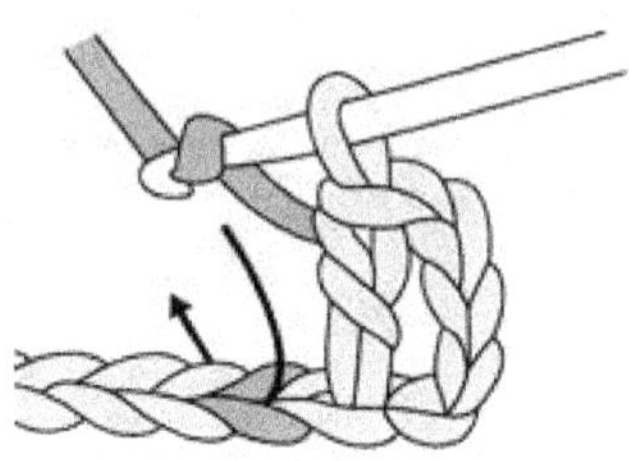

It is time to finish your first row of the double crochet and work on the dc stitch in each consecutive chain stitch crossways the base chain. It will become the foundation chain for the next chain.

There will be 16 double crochet stitches in the 1st row and count the turning chain in the first dc.

Revolve your work with the back side in front of you. It will help you to start the second row.

It will be the 3rd chain to yarn over the hook and you may chain 3 stitches for the revolving chain.

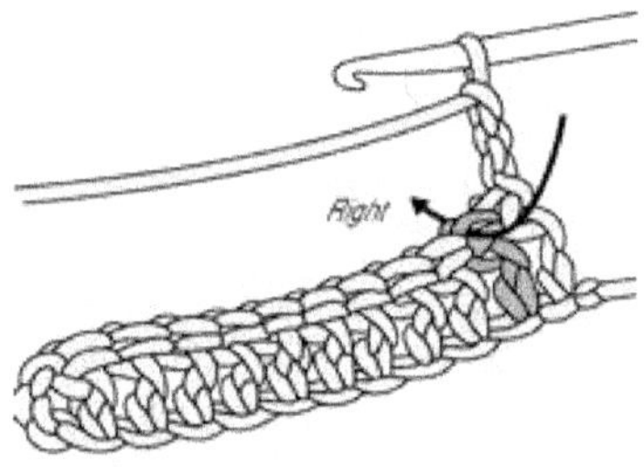

Miss the initial stitch of the row directly beneath the rotating chain, put in your fastener into the subsequent stitch.

Be careful, and don't insert the hook in the wrong place.

It is time to repeat the 3rd, 4th, and 5th steps for the next 14 dc stitches. Make sure to YO before putting on the hook in every stitch.

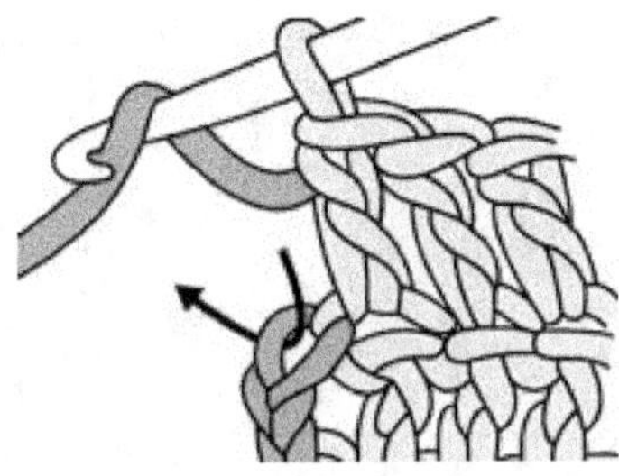

Now work 1 dc in the top chain of the preceding row's rotating chain.

Work on the 16 double crochet stitches in the 2nd row and count the turning chain as 1 dual crochet. Replicate these steps for the every extra row of double crochet. Make sure to work on the stitch until you feel comfortable.

Triple Crochet

It is also called (tr) or treble crochet and you can make long openings between the stitches. It will help you to produce loose fabric.

Now you can do the 15 chain stitches (ch 15). It is time to make your foundation chain.

You will chain 4 additional stitches and these will make turning chain.

Now YO (yarn over) the hook twice and pop in your fastener in the 5th chain from the hook.

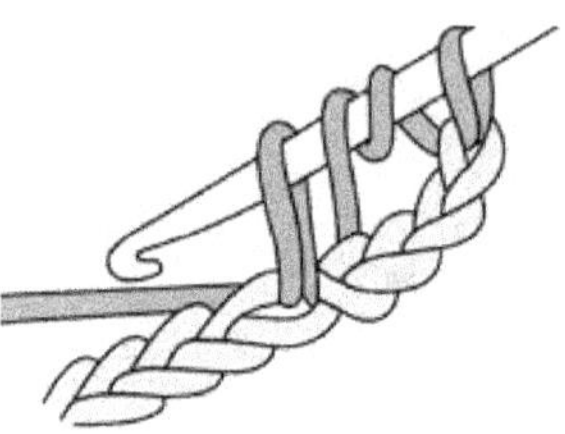

It is time to yarn over the clasp and softly pull the wrapped hook through the middle of the chain stitch, moving the wrapped yarn throughout the stitch.

You should have 4 loops on your hook.

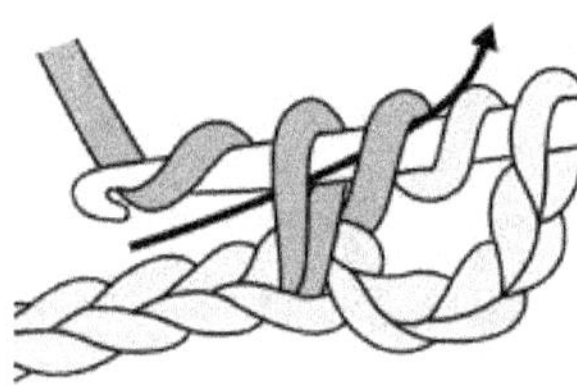

It is time to Yarn over the fastener and drag your thread throughout the initial 2 loops on your hook.

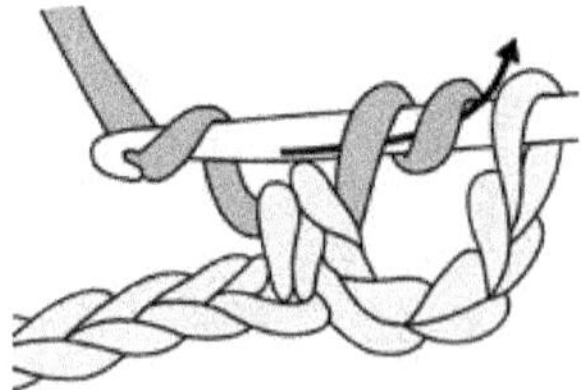

Yarn over the fastener and drag your thread through the subsequent 2 loops on your fastener.

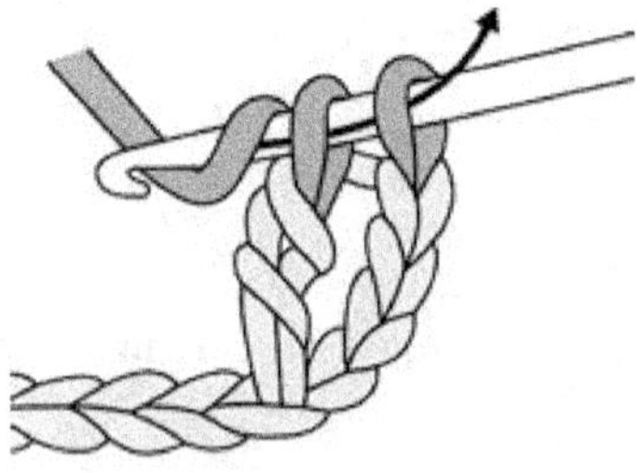

Now YO (yarn over) the fastener and drag your yarn through the preceding two loops on the hook.

One tr (triple crochet) stitch is complete and you will have one remaining loop on the hook.

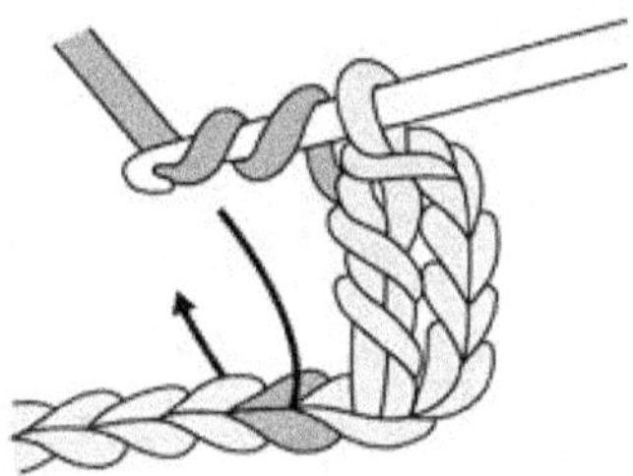

Yarn over two times and put in your fastener in the subsequent sequence of the base chain.

After this step, the row will be finished.

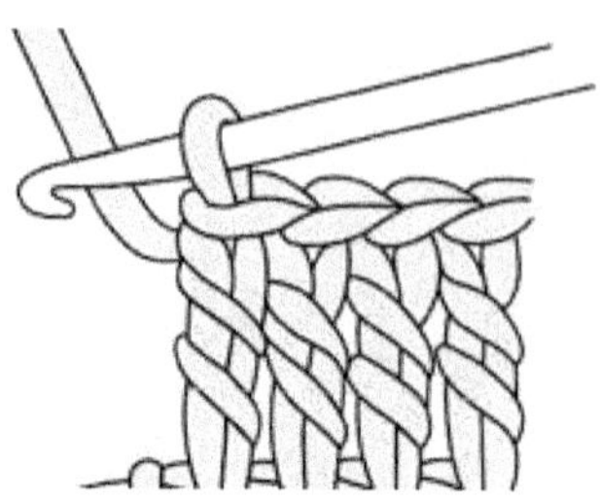

You may work on the each consecutive chain on the triple crochet in each successive chain crosswise the foundation chain.

Now there will be 16 triple crochet stitches in the first row and you need to count the turning chain as the 1st triple crochet.

Now turn your work, and you should turn the work to start the 2nd row.

Now work on the ch 4 (4th chain) and yarn over the hook twice.

Now make the stitches of the turning chain.

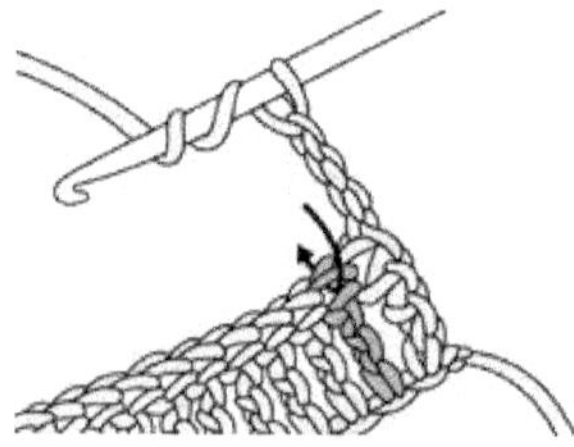

You can skip the initial stitch of the row straightly underneath the turning chain and pop in your hook in the subsequent chain.

Now skip the initial stitch and keep the stitch count consistent in every row.

Repeat the previous step in every next row of the 14 triple crochet stitches.

It is time to follow the steps by pulling the wrapped fastener throughout the middle of the chain stitch and draw your yarn through the previous two loops.

It is time to work on first triple crochet in the top chain of the preceding row of the turning chain.

There should be 16 triple crochet stitches in the 2nd row and you can repeat the preceding row from the 2nd step to get additional rows of triple crochet. Carry on your work on the triple crochet until you find it comfortable to work with this stitch.

Increase Double Crochet at the Beginning of the Row

If you want to increase the dc stitches, it can be done by adding one stitch at the beginning of the dc row. Follow this method to increase the double crochet:

Create a swatch of dc stitches.

Work on the chain 3 (ch 3).

It required the similar numbers as required for the dc turning chain. Work into the first stitch of the row such as:

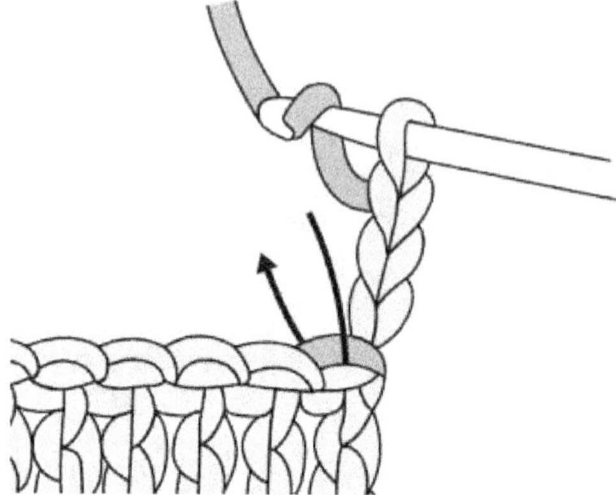

It will be under the turning chain that you typically skip. Now conclude the rest of the row through a normal procedure. Work on the 1st dc stitch in each stitch to crossways the row.

Now look at the sign used in the graphic crochet figure to represent an increase in the start of the row.

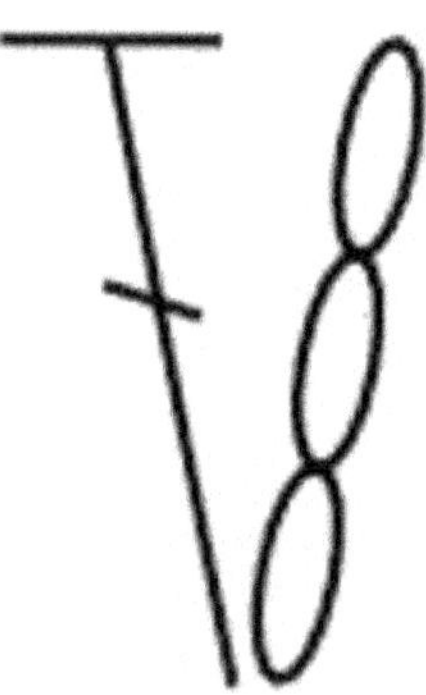

Decrease Double Crochet

The double crochet can be decreased and its abbreviation is dec and you will actually subtract the double crochet row. Decrease the stitches in the dc in the same place where you increase the stitches. You can follow the given instructions:

YO (yarn over) the hook

Pop in the hook into the next stitch and yo again.

Now drag the yarn throughout the stitch and yo

Drag the yarn throughout the initial 2 loops on the hook

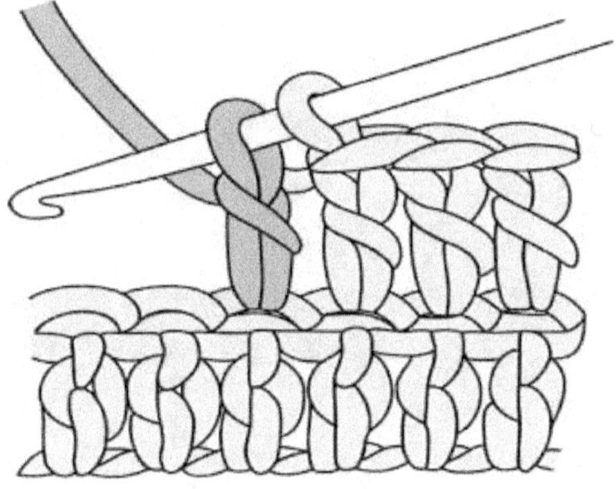

There will be two loops on the hook and you have to yarn over the hook.

Now pop in your hook into the subsequent stitch.

YO again and drag the yarn through the stitch.

YO and drag the yarn via the initial two loops on the hook.

YO and drag the yarn via all three loops on the hook.

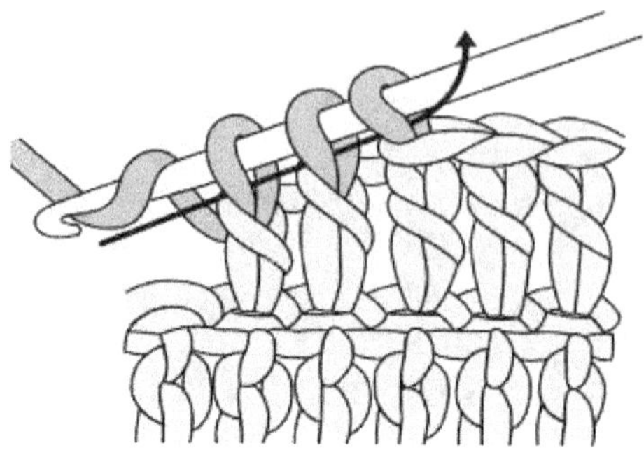

Now you will make 1 complete dc stitch and decrease it. Check the diagram to understand the crochet stitch.

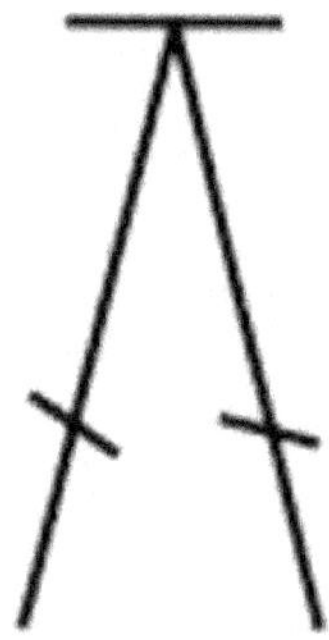

Materials

There are some main materials needed in crocheting, without them crocheting cannot be performed. Most important parts of crocheting are hook and material for crocheting. The materials that will be crocheted are usually thread, strands or yarns.

There are some other materials which play a vital role in crocheting. For example, measuring tape and gauge measure for measuring the crochet length and for counting number of stitches.

Row counter and plastic rings are used very rarely and for important projects only. Similarly, cardboard cuttings are used to make tassels and pom pom circle is used for making pom poms. In older times, only organic fibers were used for making crochet but now synthetic fibers are only used.

Crochet hooks

Crochet hooks are of different sizes and are made up of different materials like bone, aluminum, bamboo, plastic and steal. The shaft's diameter determines the sizing. A crocheter will follow the pattern to make stitches of particular sizes so that a needed thickness is reached.

If the thickness can't be reached with the help of one hook then another hook is needed till stitches reach the required size. It totally depends on the crafter to use hook of whatever material he or she wants. Crafter may prefer one type over the other due to its high aesthetic value.

Yarn

Yarn is available like balls or hanks. It can also be rolled around cones or spoons. A yarn band on the skein gives description about the weight, length, dye content and washing instructions. It is very feasible to store yarn for further use and for buying additional skeins. Yarn for the whole project should be from the single dye lot. Skeins belonging to same dye lot have the same color. Whereas, skeins from different dye lot are very different, even if they look similar. They may produce stripes during wok.

A yarn's worth is specified by numerous factors, that is loft, elasticity, washability and colorfastness, softness, durability for abrasion, fuzziness, tendency to twist, weight, blocking and felting qualities, comfort and physical appearance.

Crochet making has some benefits:

- Relaxation

Crochet is a very relaxing activity and some crochet makers consider it an antidepressant. It diverts mind from depressing activities.

- Covering

It is the most common and obvious benefit of crochet. People make scarves, blankets, sweaters, Afghans, shawls, hats etc.

- Creativity

Some people think that crochet making gives them chance to express their creativity and be creative. They show their creative idea in crochet making.

- Knowledge

Some people learn crochet and some people teach crochet. Both are the way of gaining knowledge.

Chapter 2- Lets practice making crochets!

Strand Afghan Pattern

This is the best pattern for beginners who are interested in making an afghan with 2 stranded of yarn. It's a suitable afghan for those who wish to try making a crochet in a relaxing atmosphere. This is very easy crochet to make.

Things you need:

Approximately 48 ounces beaten weight yarn
Hook – P size
A pair of scissors

Procedure:

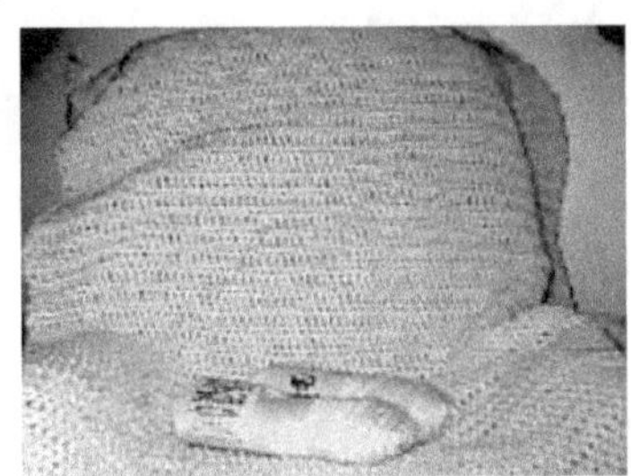Start by making the row number one. Use crochet chain 79. Put single crochet in the chain with the help of the hook and across each chain. Then start making row number two. Use crochet chain3. Now, you have to skip first single crochet. Turn double crochet in each single crochet across. Start making row number three. Turn chain crochet. Pass each single crochet across double chain. Move single chain in top of chain 3.

Now, come to edging.

Edging:

Use chain 1, you are not supposed to turn. Move 3 single chains in each corner of the pattern. Now, you have to join slip stitch to first single stitch. Fasten your yarn. Interlace in ends.

Groovy ghan

Things you must keep before getting started:

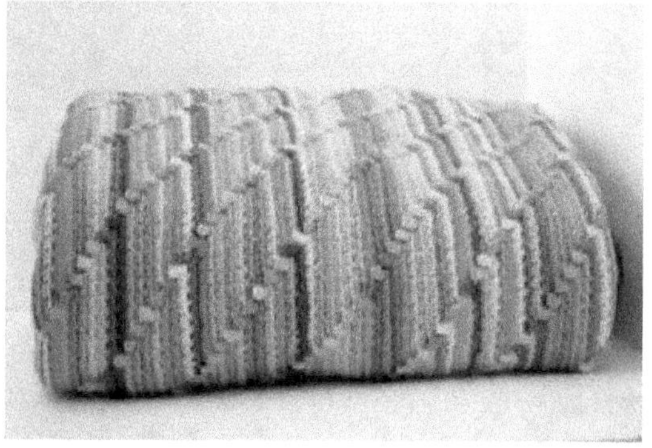

- *a crochet hook (use a 5 mm hook)*
- *yarn*
- *a pair of scissors*
- *a darning needle*

Procedure:

✓ We will start by chaining 40, 1 for turning. This will help to keep the stitch count even.

✓ Turn and make a stitch chain in every single stitch. This will be done by placing hook in the bump on the back of the chain. Chainless single crochet foundation stitch can also be used. If you are using chainless single crochet foundation stitch, use can skip the step one.

Continue this step, until the chain is completed. Cut the yarn and haul through the loop, on your hook.

✓ Make one more row of single crochet. Every single round is from right to left. Start with a standing single crochet. Making a slip knot on your hook and the single crochet should be made in the back loops only.

✓ Now let's change the color. This will make your pattern look cooler. Color will be changed from every row. New color will be started from the right hand side. We will start with the single crochet stitch. Single crochet back loops only. Now, we will start the double crochet. Put your hook in the stitch in the second row below but don't forget to use the ridge of the front loop. You will now have to make ten single crochets and front loop double crochet in the second row but it should be below. You are supposed to repeat this till the end.

✓ Now you have to change the color again.

✓ Now, change the color once more, make a positioned single crochet stitch on the right hand side and start creating crochet six times before making the front loop double crochet. Now, give a glance to your work, you will notice that you are shifting the double crochet one stitch to the left on every row, so they lie adjacent to each other! You don't to count your stitches; just single crochet in the double chain from the earlier in a circle and then make a front loop double chain subsequently after that.

If you will keep doing that in the same manner you'll sooner see the double chain's making crossways lines in your work. And this is what you need to do to make a beautiful and eye-catching crochet! Isn't that too easy?

You guys know what? You can make a baby blanket with this pattern! It sounds amazing, right? So, what are you looking at? Buy the crochet material and start making it!

Zig Zag Classic Ripple Afghan

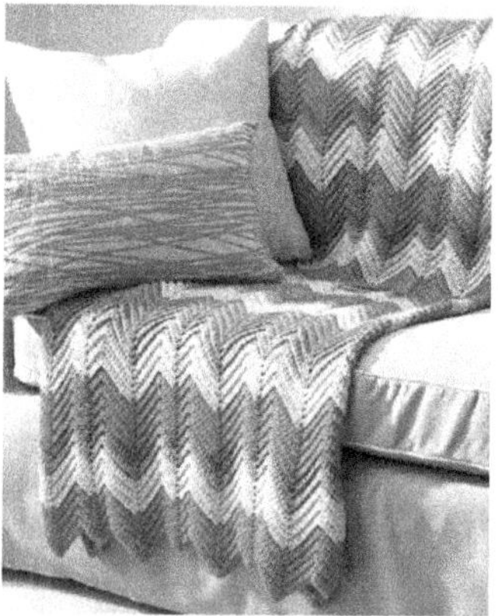

The Zig Zag Classic Ripple Afghan uses two sizes of crochet hooks and also uses medium beaten weight yarn. This pattern can be used in arranging interiors of your homes.

Mixing of yarn colors makes it ideal for home décor. It is quite amusing to know that how a simple and easy afghan pattern can change the look of your room. I must say...it gives a trendy look! Such blankets can be packed and presented as a gift to others. These are very good for laying on you sofas.

What you need?

Yarn Weight: 100kg 16 balls yarn

Hooks

A pair of scissors

Colorful yarns

Procedure:

Start by making first row. Put first single chain in second chain from the hook. Put one single chain in each of the next 9 chains. Now put each single chain in next 10 chains. You have to skip nest two chains. Pass 1 single chain from next chain. Now repeat from 1 to 9. Fasten off.

Now shift to second row. Work on back loops only. Pass 1 single crochet in each of the eight single crochets. Miss nest 2 single crochets.

We will know begin making third and fourth rows. We will start this row like second row. We will work on back loops only. Do not work the 2 single crochet. At the end, leave the last single crochet incomplete. Turn and close at the end of the 4th row.

It's to make the 5th row. Make it as the 2nd row. We will make 6th to 9th row like the 3rd row. Turn and close at the end of the 4th row. Make the 10th row as the 2nd row. Next eight rows will be similar to 3rd row.

Edging:

Join right side of crochet single crochet Afghan. Repeat for other side and fasten off.

Colorful Chevron Afghan

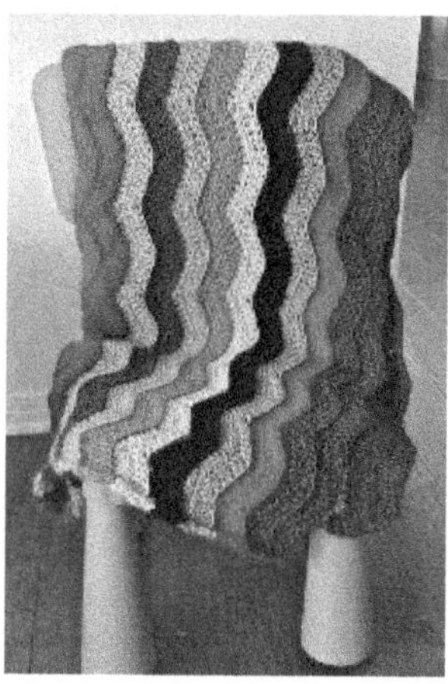

This colorful chevron Afghan is inspired by

The Missoni chevron design. You are free to use any colors. This will give a coo effect to your eyes and soul. If you want to make a similar pattern shown in the figure, you can use the stripe sequence chart. You can give your home a soothing affect by decorating with colorful crocheted afghan. It uses J hook in making.

Procedure:

Start by making the row number one. Use single chain 79. Put single crochet in the double crochet stitch with the help of the hook and across each chain. Then start making row number two. Use crochet chain 3. Now, you have to skip first single crochet.

Turn double crochet in each single crochet across so that it makes a cross. Start making row number three. Turn chain crochet. Pass each single crochet across double chain. Move single chain in top of chain 3. Turn and repeat this process. Break off.

Now come to edging.

Addicted to Chevron Afghan

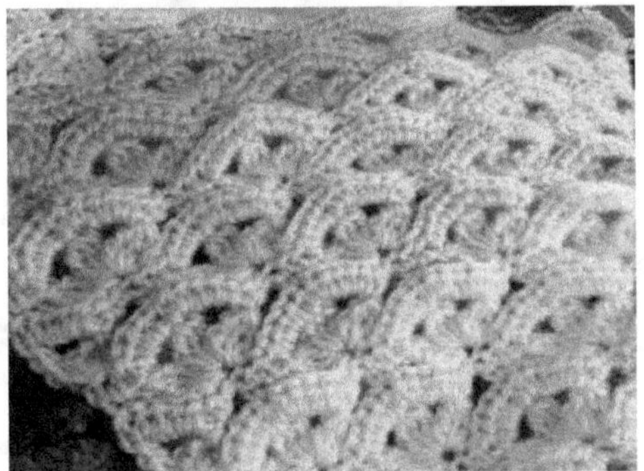

Readers! You already know Chevron is a very neat design to make. You can become addicted to it. You any two colors of the yarn. You will need four skeins. The crochet you will make will be 47 inches long and 60 inches wide. This afghan definitely gives cozy feelings. You can also make shawls with this pattern.

Irish wave baby Afghan

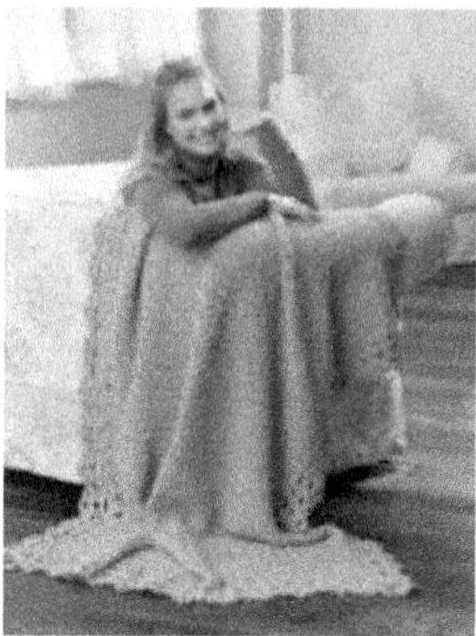

This crochet pattern will make a cozy baby blanket. The baby blanket can easily be converted into a blanket for adults. This is very simple. It can be done by increasing the number of waves. By changing the yarn weight and hook size, you can simply change the appearance and size of the Afghan.

Fireside Afghan

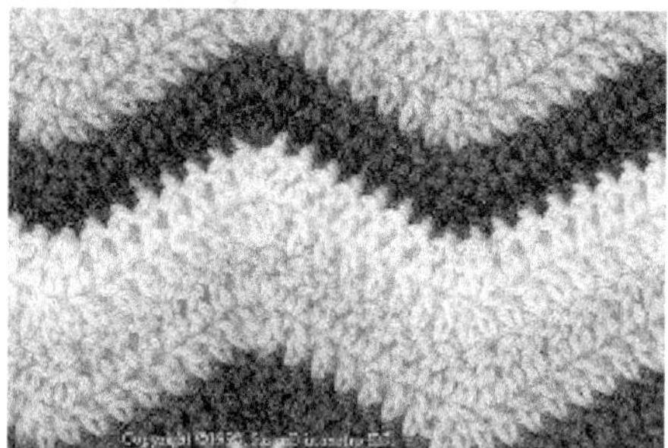

Fireside Afghan is a very unique art. It is the cross stitches that give a distinctive look the Afghan. This pattern has blocks. It is not very difficult to stitch as far as you will be following the below steps:

Things you need:

Chadwick's red heart knitting worsted

60 balls of light yellow

8 balls of wood brown for border

Afghan hook no. 6

Procedure:

This will make 49 by 67 inches blanket. Use yellow ball and make chain of ¼ inches. Make the Afghan stitch. Break it here. Attach the brown string to the corner and make 3 single crochet in the corner. You have to skip 1st chain. Repeat the first step. Make 3 single crochet in each corner. Break off. For embroidery follow some readymade pattern.

For border, you will have to make three rounds. Brown will be attached to the corner, single crochet also be attached to the corner and in each chain one, make single crochet in each corner and join. For second round, make single crochet in single chain. Make 3 single chains in center and join. For 3rd round, make 3 single chains in next single crochet. Repeat. Joint the corners and break off.

Floral Motif Afghan

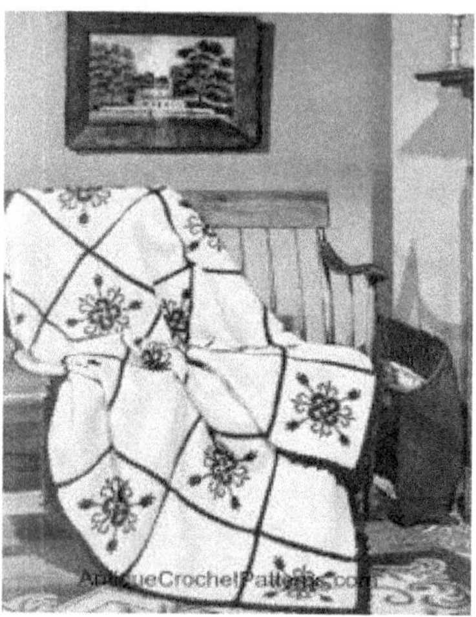

Specialized soft yarn is utilized for the making of floral motif Afghan pattern. A popcorn stitch is used for the making of this pattern. Thirty five floral motifs can be crocheted using four colors.

You can make use of the colors shown in the pictures or you can show your own creativity. This crochet helps to keep warm so it is best to be crocheted in winter.

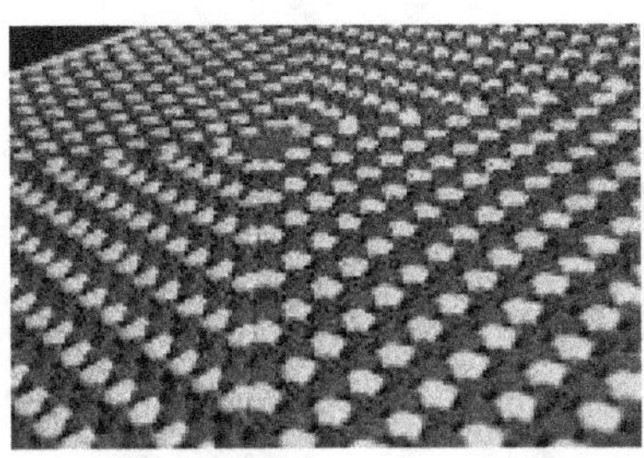

Tutti Fruiti Afghan

As the name shows this is a very colorful crochet like tutti fruiti ice-cream. Use five strands of yarn together. This will create a spiral pattern. Mostly colors like kiwi, peacock and turquoise are widely used for the preparation of this Afghan.

Candy Twist Afghan

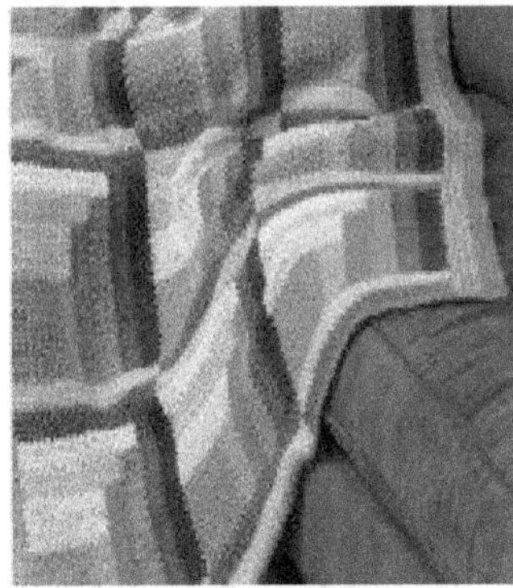

Yummy!!! Isn't your mouth watering?

Well! It's not a candy. It is a candy twist afghan. It is an exhibition of very bright and beautiful colors. It will also give you a sight of rainbow colors. You will need one skein of each color to make this afghan. Multiple colors of your choice can be used.

Finger Crochet Afghan Pattern

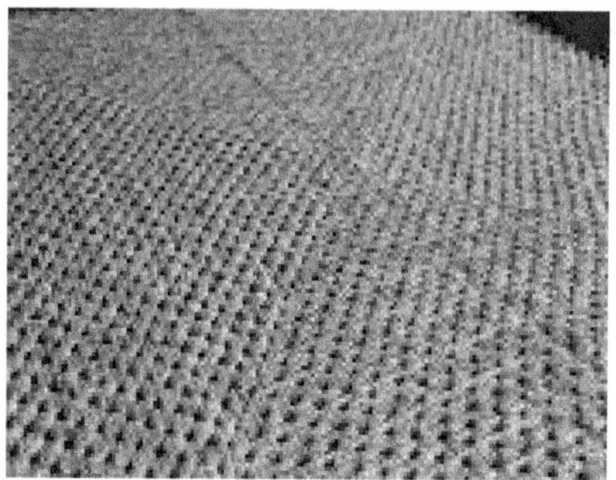

Arm knitting is a primal but finger crocheting is somewhat new-fangled. It is a process in which you have to make patterns using your fingers. This crochet is easy, even for the beginners.

Materials:

Bernat Blanket Yarn

Contrast A Vintage White 3 balls

Contrast B Silver Steel

Procedure:

Hold both the strands together. Use finger crochet technique and make four chains.

1st row: Use a single crochet in second chain from hook. Keep in mind that a single crochet should be in each chain.

2nd row: Repeat the second row until work measures approximately 56 inches Fasten off. You will notice that at the end it will form a chunky looking crochet afghan that can be snuggled throughout the winter.

Cool Crochet Long Cabin Afghan

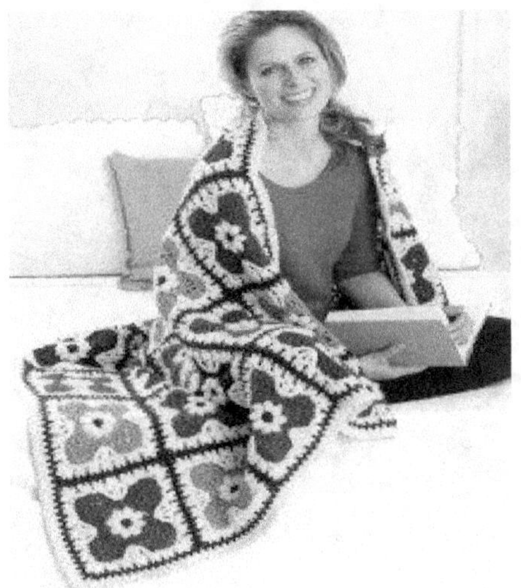

You can give a cool crochet long cabin Afghan look, to a rural pattern. This crochet afghan pattern was inspired by a traditional design but due to the addition of multiple colors, it looks classy. You can use it for warming yourself in winters.

Materials needed:

Red heart yarn (multi colors)

Hook

Yarn needles

Procedure:

This crochet will be 44 by 58. Start from working on the piece in the lower corner. The throw is usually made up of 12 squares which are arranged in 3 columns. Join each square with the previous squares. Each square will have 12 logs of colors arranged Iog quilt manner. Make all squares using larger hooks. Smaller hooks will be used for making final borders.

World's Easiest Afghan

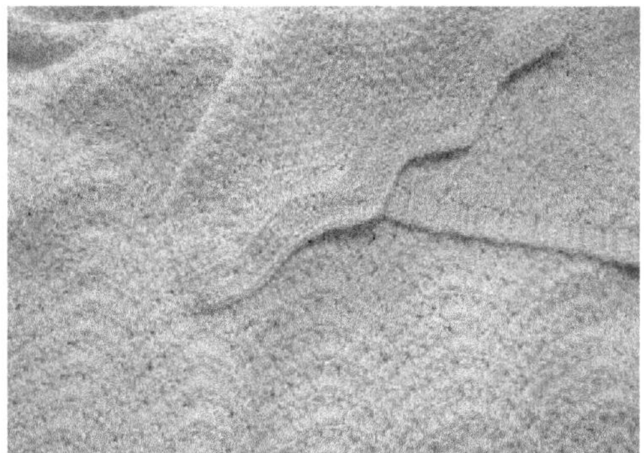

As the name shows, this is a very easy and basic Afghan. This crochet can be made by anyone. Its texture is very fascinating and unique. Dark emerald green is the option for making this type of crochet. It is bets for kid's room and living room as it brighten up the colors of the surroundings.

Things you need:

Crochet hook

Yarn

Procedure:

Pass the 1st single crochet in 2nd chain from the hook. Pass 1st double chain in next chain. Repeat from the end. For second row, pass single crochet in 1st double chain. Then, pass 1st double chain in next single crochet. Repeat from the end and turn .Repeat 2nd row until a 152.5 cm blanket is formed.

Blush Rose Afghan

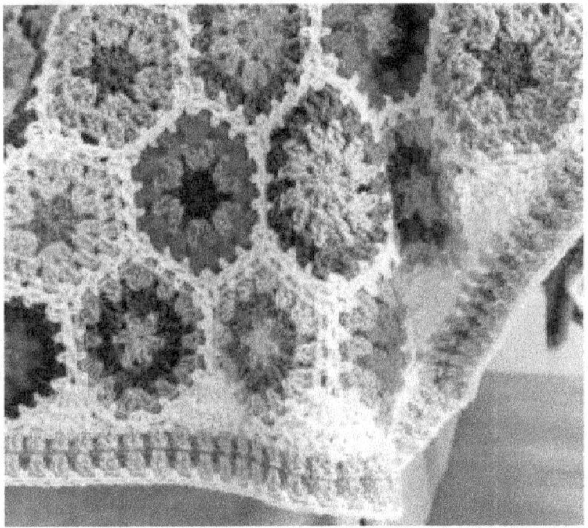

This beautiful Blush Rose Afghan is mostly used and loved by the ladies. You can easily carry this crochet to the parks and picnics.

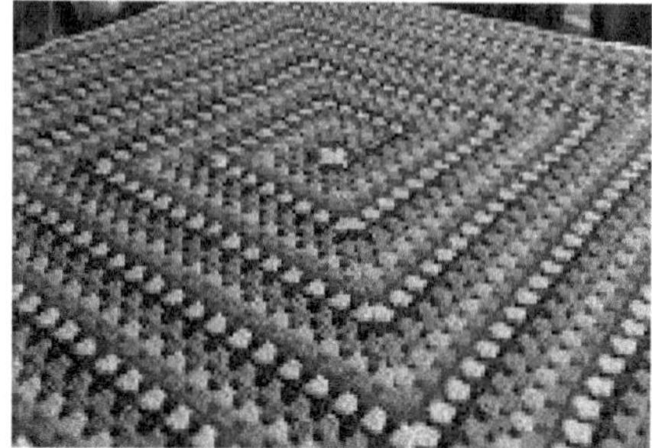

Granny Hexagon Afghan

This is a very a different granny afghan as compared to typical afghans. Its unique   shapes and funny patterns create a stunning design. This will give a bubbling effect to your home. Hexagons give a floral look to your home.

Granny square crochet pattern

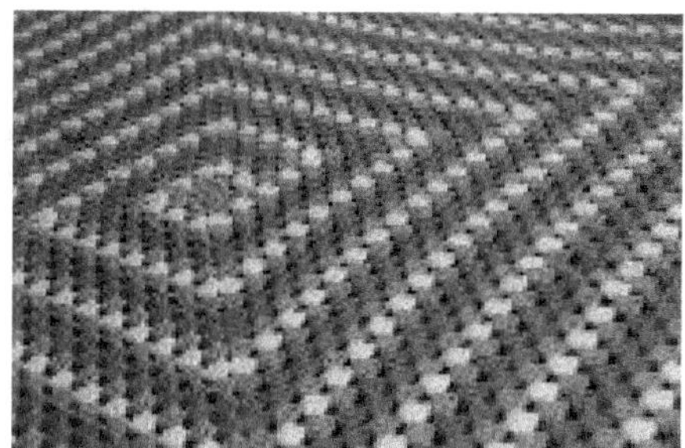

Granny square crochet patterns can be of large importance for armatures to work on especially if there is one strand of yarn available to work with. Some people like working with tremendous soft yarns while others like a more rough yarn with that little bit of extra texture to it.

American Afghan

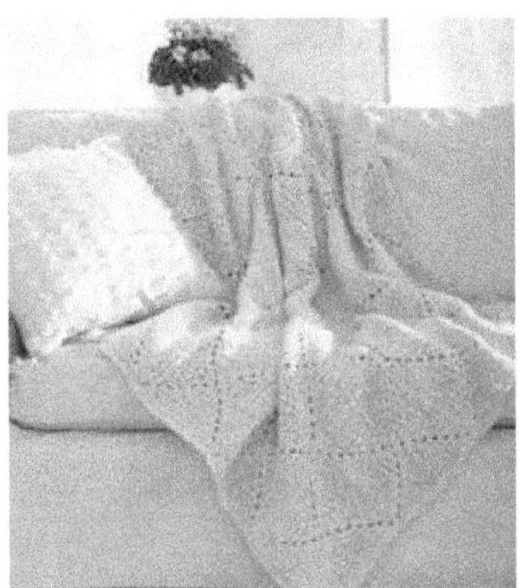

Patriotic American Afghan is made by using red and blue colors. This is a grand crochet to carry during the months of August and July. American Afghan crochet can be given as a gift to someone in the Army.

Neutral Crochet Ripple Afghan

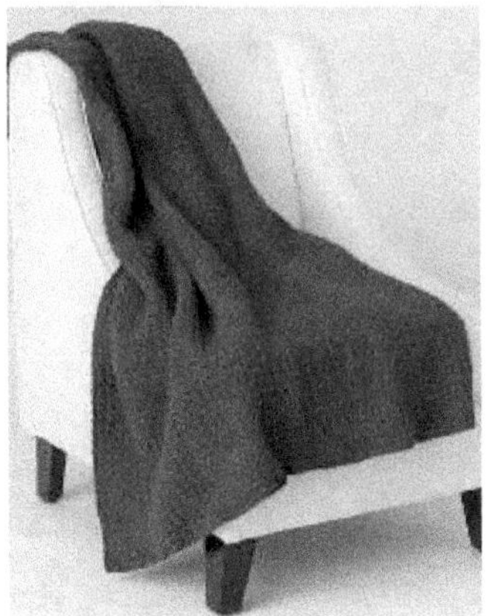

The crochet ripple afghan pattern is all about elegant colours and fancy ornaments. It works in single crochet for a warm cover.

Crochet hook 5mm

Yarn 4

Procedure:

1st row: Make 1st chain by putting it in the single chain. Put 1st single chain in each of next 8 chains. 3 single crochet in next chain. Put 1st single crochet in each of next 9 chains. Skip next 2 chains. Turn.

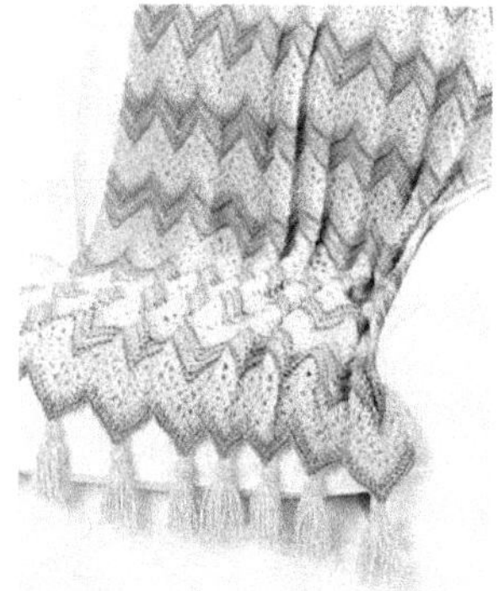

2nd row: Working in back loops only.

3rd row: Working in back loops only

4th and 5th rows: repeat 1st and 2nd row.

6th, 7th and 8th row: Skip first single crochet. Put 1st double crochet in next single crochet. Skip next 2 single crochet. Repeat and turn. Fasten off.

9th row: As 8th row.

V Stitch Crochet Ripple Afghan

V stitch crochet ripple afghan is made up of five colours that will give a cozy look to our room. Working v stitch crochet afghan is a good way to refresh your home decor by just blending some colours. The V stitches in this crochet afghan pattern produce a lacy, open design that will fit with any home.

Foolproof Afghan

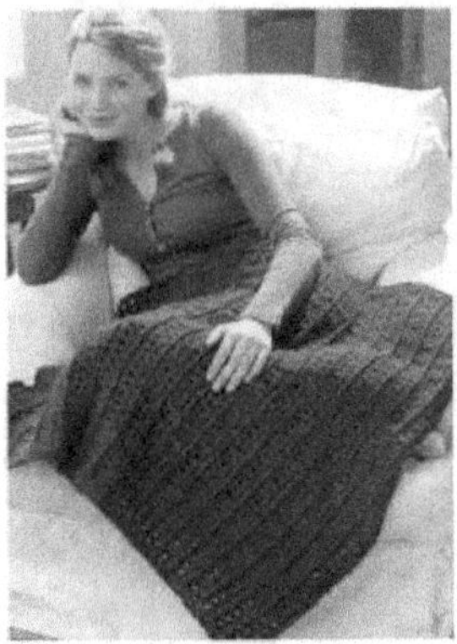

If you are looking for a easy crochet pattern that you can work upon and at the same time do you're other tasks, then foolproof Afghan is the best option for you. This crochet is easy to make for everybody.

You are going to use front post of double crochet. This will give the afghan, a smooth texture. You will love having it at your homes especially in cold weather.

Soft Clusters Ripple Afghan

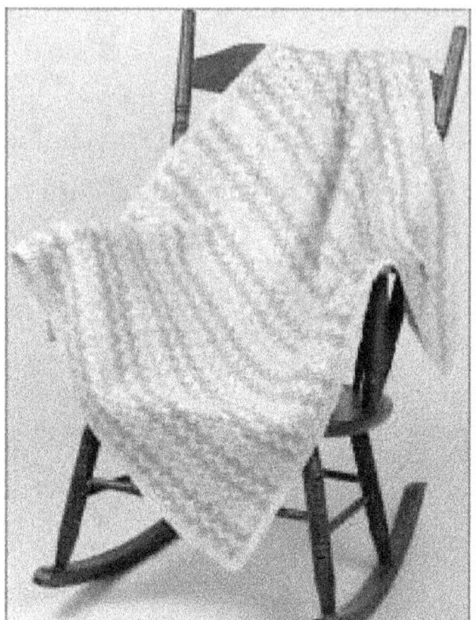

What's good about this one is the fact that boundaries can be made as you want them to. Ripple pattern is quite easy in making. It can be done in any variations of colors. Soft beaten yarn can make this afghan extremely soft.

Zigzag Shells Baby Afghan

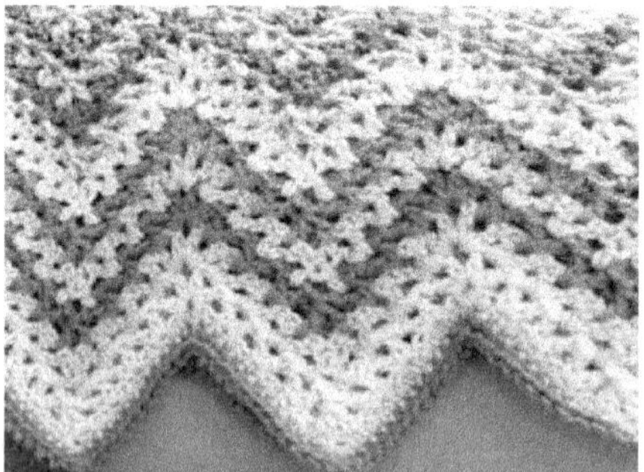

This is a very delicate crochet pattern. It has a very delicate pattern. It is made by a G size hook. As the name indicates, this is used by babies as a blanket. Its size is 35 by 45 inches.

Chapter 3 – Crochet Afghans Simple Patterns

There are some simple patterns that can be followed to make crochet Afghans:

Afghan Crochet Square

- • Completed Size: 12" square

- Size "H" crochet hook

Follow the Pattern:

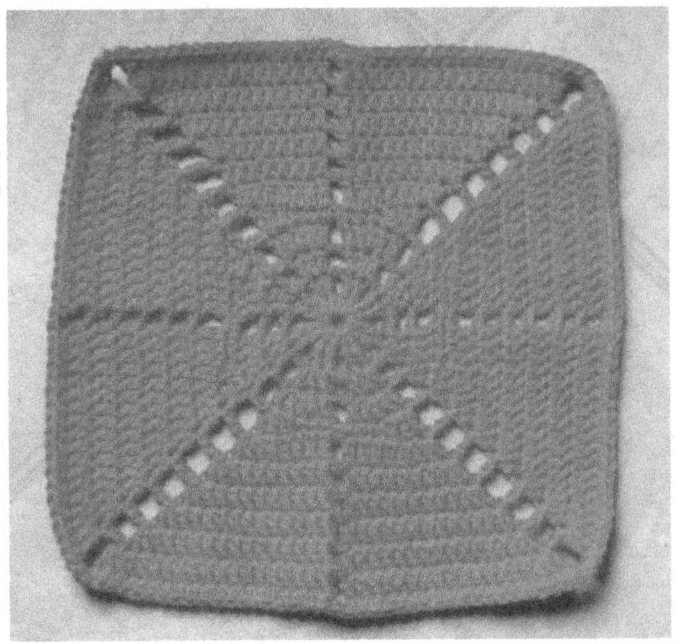

ch 4.

Row 1: (triple stitch) tr in 4th ch from your hook, it is time for ch2,* (2tr, ch2), replicate from * 6 times, now slip stitch to top ch4.

Row 2: In this row, you will do ch3, 2dc in subsequent tr and ch2,* ((double crochet) dc in consequent tr and 2dc in succeeding tr, ch2), replicate from * almost 6 times, and slip stitch to top of ch3 before starting the third one.

Row 3: the row will start with ch3, now 3dc in subsequent dc, and dc in subsequent dc, it is time for ch2, * now dc in subsequent dc (double crochet), 3dc in subsequent dc (double crochet), dc in subsequent dc, and ch2, replicate from * around, now slip stitch in top of ch3.

Row 4: in this row, you will start with ch3 and 2edc (extended double crochet) in subsequent dc (double crochet), sc in subsequent 3 dc (double crochet), sc in subsequent ch2 sp, sc in subsequent 3 dc, 2edc in next dc, dc in next dc, ch3,* dc in subsequent dc, 2edc in subsequent dc, sc in next 3 dc, sc in subsequent ch2 sp, sc in subsequent 3 dc, 2edc in subsequent dc, dc in subsequent dc, ch3, replicate from * around and slip stitch to top of ch3.

Row 5: It is time to work again ch3 and 2dc in alike stitch as beg ch, dc in subsequent 5 sts, ch2, skip subsequent sc, dc in subsequent 5 sts and 3dc in subsequent st, ch3, * 3dc in subsequent st, dc in subsequent 5 sts, ch2, skip subsequent sc, dc in subsequent 5 sts, 3dc in subsequent st, ch3, replicate from * around and slip stitch to top of ch3 before working on the subsequent line.

Row 6: ch3 and 2dc in same sp (space) as beg ch and dc (double crochet) in subsequent 7 sts, ch2, skip ch2 sp, dc in next 7 sts, 3dc in subsequent st, * ch3, 3dc in another st, dc in next 7 sts and ch2, leave out ch2 sp and dc in subsequent 7 sts and 3dc in subsequent st, replicate from * around, and now slip stitch to top of ch3 before the next line.

Row 7: It will be ch3 and 2dc in similar sp as implore ch, dc in subsequent 9 dc and ch2, miss out ch2 sp and dc in subsequent 9 dc and 3dc in subsequent dc, * ch3, 3dc in subsequent dc, dc in subsequent 9 dc, ch2, skip ch2 sp, dc in subsequent 9 dc, 3dc in subsequent dc, replicate from * around and slip stitch to top of beg ch3.

Row 8: you will start with ch3 and 2dc in similar sp as beg ch, dc in subsequent 11 dc, ch2, skip ch2 sp, dc in subsequent 11 dc, 3dc in subsequent dc, * ch3 and 3dc in subsequent dc and dc in subsequent 11 dc, ch2, skip ch2 sp, dc in subsequent 11 dc, 3dc in next dc, replicate from * around, slip stitch to top of beg ch3.

Row 9: ch3, 2dc in similar sp as beg ch, dc in subsequent 13 dc, ch2, skip ch2 sp, dc in subsequent 13 dc, 3dc in subsequent dc, * ch3, 3dc in subsequent dc, dc in subsequent 13 dc, ch2, skip ch2 sp, dc in subsequent 13 dc, 3dc in subsequent dc, replicate from * around, slip stitch to top of beg ch3 before starting the next line.

Row 10: ch1, sc in every stitch located around, along with 1sc in ch2 sp, and 3sc in corner sps, slip stitch to top of beg ch3. Tie up to secure the stitches.

Extended Double Crochet

YO (yarn over) and insert the hook subsequent stitch or chain and YO and pull up the ring and yarn over and draw through 1 loop. It will make one chain and now yarn over and pull via 2 loops to complete 1 edc.

- V-stitch: (dc, ch 2, dc) in designated ch sp or between 2 stitches designated.

- Shell: (2 dc, ch 2, 2 dc) in designated ch sp.

- Color A: Turqua

- Color B: White

- Color C: Light Teal

Follow the pattern:

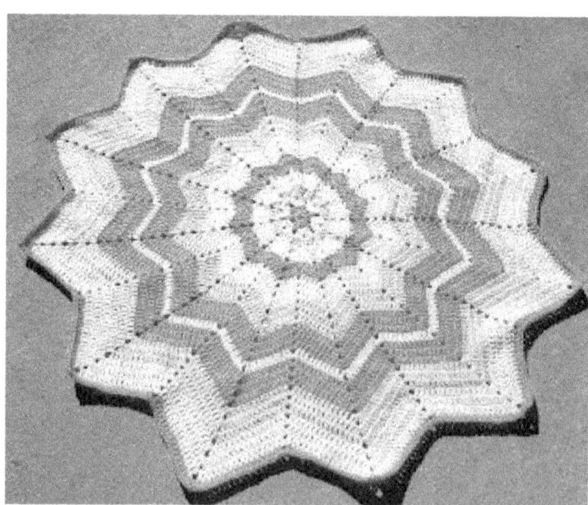

It is time to use color A ch 4 and join with a slip st in 4th ch from closure to make a ring.

Round 1: Ch 3, dc in ring, ch 2, *(2 dc, ch 2) repeat from * 4 more times in ring; join with a slip st in the top of beginning ch-3. Finish it. (12 dc, 6 ch-2)

Round 2: Using color B join with a slip st in any ch-2 sp, ch 3, (dc, ch 2, 2 dc) in similar sp, ch 1, *(shell, ch 1) in ch-2 sp, replicate from * around; unite with slip st in top of beginning ch-3. Conclude off. (24 dc, 6 ch-1 sps, 6 ch-2 sps)

Round 3: Now you can use color C unite with a slip st in one ch sp, ch 3, (dc, ch 2, 2 dc) in similar ch sp, *casing in next ch sp, replicate from * around; unite with a slip st in the top of beg ch-3. Finish off. (48 dc, 12 ch-2 sps). It is time to start the next row.

Round 4: Using color B join with a slip st in 2nd dc of any shell, ch 3, shell in ch-2 sp, dc in next st, sk following 2 sts, *dc in following st, shell in ch-2 sp, dc in next st, sk next 2 sts, repeat from * around; join with a slip st in top of beg ch-3. (72 dc, 12 ch-2 sps)

Round 5: Slip st into next st, ch 3, dc in next st, *V-st in next ch-2 sp, dc in following 2 sts, omit following 2 sts, dc in following 2 sts, replicate from * and around, sk preceding 2 sts; connect with slip st in top of the beginning ch-3. Close off. (72 dc, 12 ch-2 sps). Proceed to next step.

Important Note:

In all rounds, you can change the yarn color and unite new color with the slip stitch. One stitch to the left of the slip stitch and you can complete by joining the last round mutually and then finish it.

If you want to start with a new color of yarn, you will work in the round in back loops right through the round. After changing the initial yarn color, you can work with both loops and change the color of the yarn once again.

Round 6: With the help of color A, you can unite with a slip st single stitch to the left of the slip st to work in the back loop throughout, ch 3, dc in BL of subsequent st, *shell in next ch-2 space, dc in BL of following 2 sts, sk 2 sts, dc in BL of following 2 sts, replicate from * and around, sk preceding 2 sts; unite with slip st in top of beginning ch-3. (96 dc, 12 ch-2 sps). It is time for 7th row.

Round 7: Slip st into next st, ch 3, dc in next 2 sts, *shell in next ch-2 sp, dc in next 3 sts, skip 2 sts, dc in next 3 sts, replicate from * around, sk preceding 2 sts; unite with slip st in top of beginning ch-3. (120 dc, 12 ch-2 sps)

Round 8: Slip st in a subsequent st, ch 3, dc in the subsequent 3 sts, *V-st in subsequent ch-2 sp, dc in subsequent 4 sts, sk 2 sts and dc in subsequent 4 sts, replicate from * around, sk previous 2 sts; unite with slip st in top of beg ch-3. (120 dc, 12 ch-2 sps)

Round 9: Slip st in a subsequent st, ch 3, dc in a subsequent 3 sts, *shell in next ch-2 sp, dc in subsequent 4 sts, sk 2 sts, dc in subsequent 4 sts, replicate from * around, sk last 2 sts; join with slip st in top of beg ch-3. (144 dc, 12 ch-2 sps)

Round 10: Slip st in next st, ch 3, dc in next 4 sts, *shell in next ch-2 sp, dc in next 5 sts, sk 2 sts, dc in next 5 sts, replicate from * around, sk last 2 sts; join with slip st in top of beg ch-3. (168 dc, 12 ch-2 sps)

You can continue this pattern by repeating different rounds and always start with V-st for the first round and a shell for the second round. Repeat 8, 9 and 10 round to make a smooth blanket.

Chapter 4 – What is the Tunisian crochet?

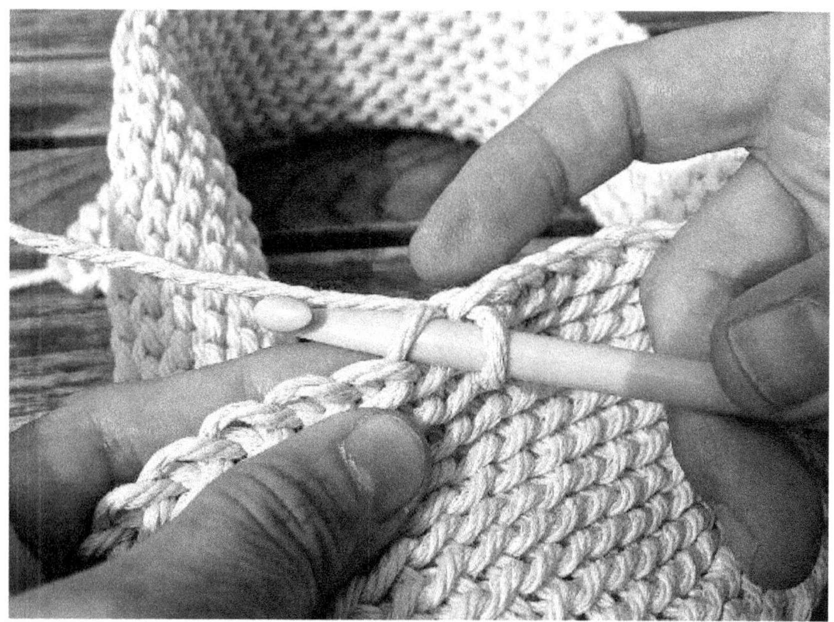

If you love crocheting, you will definitely love the Tunisian crochet, which represents a unique blend between crochet and knitting. Even though its origins are not exactly known, this type of crocheting has become more and more popular in the past few years, due to the fact that it allows for the creation of a distinct fabric. The technique leads to a woven aspect, instead of the traditional knitted or crocheted appearance.

In order to begin your Tunisian crocheting adventure, you will require an elongated hook, which has a stopper at its end. This is known as an Afghan hook and it resembles the knitting needle, as it has a stopper as well as the end. The purpose of the stopper is to prevent the stitches that are held on the tool from falling off.

The Tunisian crochet is distinct from the standard crocheting technique, in the sense that each row has two different passes. On one hand, you have the forward pass, in which the created loops are maintained around the hook. On the other hand, there is the reverse pass, in which the loops are backed off the respective hook. Apart from that, it is a known fact that the Tunisian crochet does not require for the work to be turned. This is the reason why the fabric's right side is permanently going to represent the facing side.

Because the Tunisian crochet uses the Afghan hook, it is also known as the Afghan crochet or stich. The Afghan hook is necessary for this type of crocheting, allowing you to complete a wide range of patterns and stitches. As you will have the opportunity to see below, the stitch or pattern created depends on the method of hook insertion, as well as on how the working yarn has been held. The various Tunisian stitches that can be created are beautiful to say the least.

As you will have the opportunity to discover, the fabrics that you are going to create with the Tunisian crochet is not as elastic as the one obtained with other types of crocheting.

Moreover, it is considerably thicker, especially when it comes to the knit stitch. Because of these properties, the Tunisian crochet is recommended for the making of thick blankets, as well as for other winter knits. On the other hand, you might find it difficult to create items such as babywear or socks using this crocheting technique.

It is a known fact that the fabric created with the help of the Tunisian crochet has curling tendencies, which means that its final shape is obtained with the help of the blocking process. This process entails either the wetting or the steaming of the completed fabric, so that it has a pleasant aspect and maintains its form.

Many people are interested in learning this crocheting technique, due to the fact that it can be used to create beautiful fabrics, in a shorter period of time (in comparison to the normal crochet). If you were to compare the time of the regular crochet and the one required for the Tunisian crochet, you would discover that the latter would be half of the first one.

The Tunisian crochet is appreciated all over the world for its beautiful texture, create by the density and fluidity of the fabric. As it was already mentioned, this method of crocheting cannot be mistaken for the traditional crochet.

This is because, in the traditional crochet, you complete a row of stitches and, then, you turn the work. Once you have achieved that, you can move on to the next row. With the Tunisian crochet, each row requires the alternation of forward and backward passes (plus, turning the work is not required).

As you will complete your very first rows of traditional Tunisian crochet, you will begin to observe that the fabric appears woven on the right side. As for the other side, this will have a wave-like appearance. Do not be scared, thinking that this type of crochet might be too difficult for you. On the contrary, once you familiarize yourself with the basics, you will discover that it is quite simple. There are varied stitches to try out, with different color effects to be enjoyed.

Like other types of crocheting, the more you practice, the more experienced you are going to become. You can start with a practice row base and continue with stripes, as these are the easiest to make. For many people, the Tunisian crochet starts out as an interest but it turns to be more than a hobby, once they discover how many possible stitches and patterns there are.

If you are interested in practicing the Tunisian crochet, you should prepare yourself for some shopping. Start looking at the different types and colors of yarns, enjoying the number of available choices. Also, you can shop for Afghan hooks, taking advantage of the diversity offered. Keep in mind that you can create fashionable items with the help of the Tunisian crochet, so you can always take your passion to the next level.

Tunisian crochet tools

It is possible to use normal hooks for the Tunisian crochet but you should make sure that the shaft does not widen in the middle. However, for the majority of the patterns of the Tunisian crochet, you will have to use an Afghan hook. As you will have the opportunity to see for yourself, Tunisian hooks have a length of approximately 30 cm (if you are using cables, then they are even longer).

One of the most popular types of Tunisian crochets is the one that has a stopper. This is quite similar to the straight-knitting needle, however, instead of having a point at the end, it has a hook. The purpose of the stopper is to keep the stitches on the Tunisian hook. This type of crocheting needle has a length of 30 cm, which makes it suitable for the making of scarves and other similar knitwear (e.g.: shawls).

Another alternative is the double-ended Tunisian hook, which, as the name clearly points out, has hooks on both of its sides. These can be used in a similar manner as the Tunisian hook with the stopper, but you will have to be a little bit more attentive (or else you will lose your stitches). The advantage of the double-ended Tunisian hook is that you can work the Tunisian crochet in the round as well.

The Tunisian hook with extension can also be used for this type of crocheting. The advantage of these hooks is that you can attach a cord to them, of varied length, in order to make them longer (from 15 cm to 1.5 m). In a way, this type of crocheting needle resembles the interchangeable needles, the hook representing the actual difference. At the end of the cable, there is the stopper, its purpose being to prevent the stitches from falling off.

If you are not sure which type of purchase, try to think about your budget. In the situation that your budget is limited, you should go with the double-ended Tunisian crochet.

As it was mentioned above, these have a similar use as the one with the stopper but they will also give you the opportunity to work in the round (provided you desire to do so). If you are willing to spend a higher amount of money, then choose the interchangeable hooks.

These have a lighter weight, they are easier to use and they are made from various materials. If you will purchase them in sets, you will also benefit from a discounted price.

The basic length for the Tunisian hook is of 30 cm, as it has been clearly pointed out. However, it is recommended that you should always choose a hook that is two times bigger than the size indicated for a specific yarn weight.

As for the yarn, you can go with yarn DK or even heavier. You can also purchase it in two colors, as you will have to learn how to change colors as well. For working in two colors, you can always go with the double-ended hooks. Light colors are definitely recommended, as they will allow you to better see the stitches or patterns you have created.

As the Tunisian crochet has become more and more popular in the past few years, it should come as no surprise that there is a wide range of hooks to be purchased.

These hooks are made from a wide range of materials, such as bamboo, plastic, wood and aluminum. Their shape varies, allowing each person who is passionate about crocheting to choose according to personal preferences.

Keep in mind that the Tunisian crochet can cause stress on the hand and muscles of the wrist. The repetitive motion can be eliminated by choosing cabled hooks, as these are lightweight and have a guaranteed reduced effort. With these types of hooks, you can enjoy your crocheting for a prolonged period of time, without worrying about your hands or wrists.

These are the basic tools that you will require for your Tunisian crochet adventure. Once you have everything gathered, you can proceed towards learning the amazing patterns and stitches that can be created. Enjoy!

Chapter 5 – Beginning Projects for Tunisian Crochet

There is nowhere better to start than at the beginning. These projects are for those who are in the very early learning stages. Remember that you need to take it slow, and that these are for practice with a cause.

That means that they are not going to be perfect on the outset, and they may not be used for much around your house, but they are going to give you a feel for the craft, and with practice you will be making projects more advanced than these and with even more flair.

New Beginnings Shawl

Use your Tunisian crochet hook and white and green yarn.

Chain 25, and cast on these stitches onto your Tunisian crochet hook. Single crochet in each stitch across the row, creating a forward pass. Return pass doing the same. Make sure that your tension is even, and that you aren't pulling too hard on the yarn as you are working.

Repeat this pattern until you have a strip that is about 4 feet long. Tie off and switch to the other color.

Chain 25, then cast on these stitches onto your Tunisian crochet hook. Single crochet in each stitch. Return pass the same way as you did the forward pass, and repeat this until you have a strip that is about 4 feet long.

Repeat this pattern with the same color once more, then for the last time with the other color.

You are now going to have 4 strips, 2 of each of the two colors. Use your yarn needles and sew these strips together, then use your crochet hook to finish a border around the entire project.

Tie off, and if you want to make more of a hippie feel to it, make a fringe of the two colors and string them along the bottom of the shawl.

Simple Beaded Pillow

Start with your foundation chain, and chain a length of 18 inches. Now, make the first row as we talked about in the first chapter. When you are all the way across the row, simply continue up with the next row.

Go back and forth this way until you have a length of fabric that is 18 inches wide by 22 inches long.

Tie it off, then fold the fabric you have made so there is an 18 inch square, with 4 inches extra hanging off of one end.

Sew all the way up both sides, then stuff the pillow from the top. Finally, sew the seam closed along the top. Let the flap fall down over one side of the pillow, then add a button loop where it falls.

Sew a big button onto the flap, then use this button to secure the flap down. Tie off any loose ends and that's it!

Granny Square Blanket

Follow the simple pattern for the squares that we have provided, making then 6 inches wide by 6 inches long. When you have 36 of these squares, take a yarn needle and sew them together.

Take a standard crochet hook (or use your Tunisian crochet hook) and sew a border around the entire border. This is a really simple project, but it is perfect for blankets, baby showers, or anything else that you need simplicity combined with beauty.

Cross Knit Washcloth

For this project, you need to make sure you are using cotton yarn. You can use what you would like for the other projects, but as this one needs to be in water from time to time, it is important that you use a fiber that will be able to handle it.

Acrylic doesn't absorb water very well, so cotton is definitely a better option.

Make a foundation chain roughly 6 inches long, and make your first row. Work your way up the sides. Make sure your tension is even and that you are keeping the yarn firm, then tie it off firmly when you are done.

Crochet a border around the top and sides of it, then tie off that border as well. You are now ready to use your washcloth!

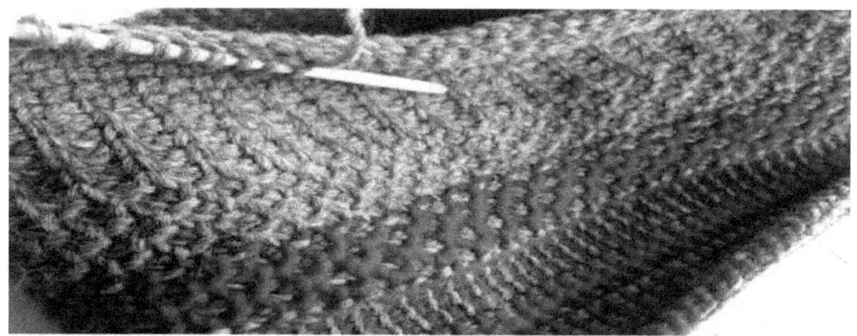

Simple Scarf

This is a pattern that uses both regular crochet and Tunisian crochet. It is relatively easy to do, but you need to pay attention to make sure you stay on the right pattern.

For starters, make a foundation chain that is about 5 inches wide. Tunisian crochet 3 rows, then chain two at the end of the third row. Turn, then double crochet for three rows. This time, don't turn the project, and do 3 more rows of the Tunisian crochet.

Add fringe to both edges, then tie off. This is a heavier scarf, even if you make it out of light yarn, so it is difficult for this scarf to be purely fashion. If you want an even warmer scarf, you can make it out of wool.

Chapter 6 – Tunisian crochet stitches

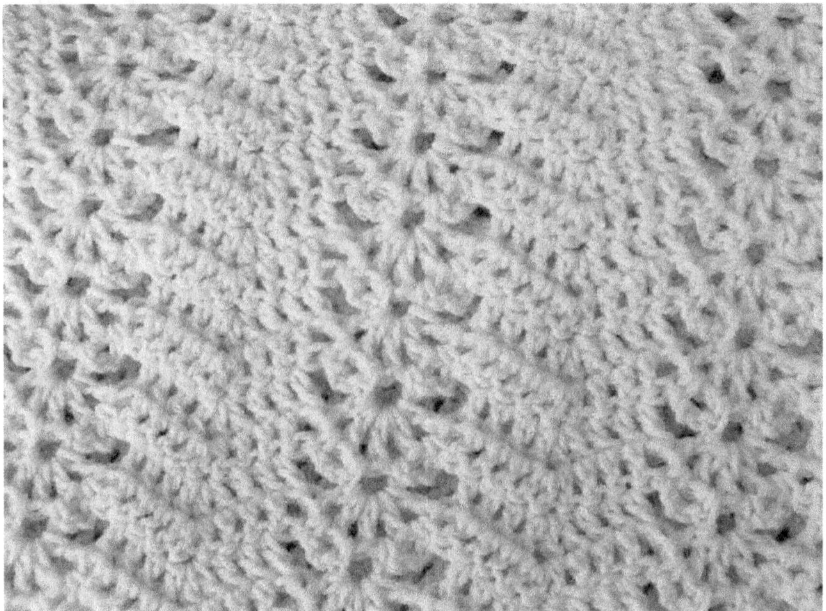

The Tunisian crochet is considered a unique form of crocheting, especially since the stitches made by hand cannot be reproduced with the help of a machine. The interesting thing is that it is also reversible, which means that each side will reveal a different pattern. Let us discover 15 of the most popular stitches out there!

#1 Tunisian simple stitch (TSS)

In order to perform the Tunisian simple stitch, you will have to slide the hook, so that it appears right at the back of the front vertical stitch. You will also have to make sure that the hook is kept at the front of the work. Then, yarn round hook and bring up a loop. Always maintain the loop on the hook.

#2 Tunisian reverse stitch (TRS)

For the Tunisian reverse stich, you will have drop the yarn in the foreground of the work. You need to make sure that it falls between the stitch that is already present on the hook and the following stitch (the one that will be picked up).

Then, slide the hook, so that it appears right at the back of the front vertical stitch (as you have done for the Tunisian simple stitch). Once you have achieved that, bring the yarn posteriorly. Yarn round hook and bring up a loop. By doing this, you will realize a sort of a knot, in the foreground of the stitch.

#3 Tunisian moss stitch (TMS)

The Tunisian moss stitch will allow to create the honeycomb pattern. In order to realize this, you will have to work one Tunisian simple stitch, followed by the Tunisian reverse stitch. Basically, you alternate them across each row of the work. However, you should make sure that, on the next row, the stitches are positioned above their counterparts.

This particular stitch is recommended for the situation when you are using two colors and you want to obtain a beautiful pattern. By placing the stitches above each other, you will realize a contrasting decoration.

#4 Tunisian purl stitch (TPS)

For the Tunisian purl stitch, you will have to incline the work in your direction. Glance past the superior margin, in order to identify the posterior vertical section of the stitch. Then, slide the hook as in the Tunisian simple stitch, making sure that it is maintained in the background of the fabric.

Yarn round hook and bring up a loop. A word of advice: do not work all of the fabric only with the simple stitch and purl stitch, as it will curl. It is recommended that you alternate the simple stitch/reverse stitch with the simple stitch/purl stitch, within the same row or at each additional row. Curling can also be prevented by using a larger hook.

#5 Tunisian knit stitch (TKS)

For the Tunisian knit stitch, the hook has to be inserted between the anterior and posterior vertical part of the stitch. Yarn round hook, then bring up a loop. Keep in mind that this type of stitch will lead to a thick fabric, which also requires a larger hook to be used. Even though this fabric might appear to be stretchy, you will see that the work is actually shorter, in comparison to the rows created with other stitches (the hook is of the same size).

#6 Tunisian full stitch (TFS)

For the Tunisian full stitch, the hook has to be inserted from the anterior to the posterior part of the work, right between the two stitches. For the first row, you will have to work between the first and second stitch.

You will also have to make sure that the distance amid the last two stitches will not be worked. In the situation that you do not compensate for the space working, you will discover that your work has inclined towards one side (growing with one stitch for each of the created rows).

#7 Tunisian extended stitch (TES)

The Tunisian extended stitch allows you to add height to each row. For this stitch, at the top of each loop, you will have to add one chain stitch. This will have to be performed for all of the stitches that are present on the row, including the first and the last one. This is the perfect stitch, in the situation that you want to create a looser fabric.

#8 Tunisian double crochet (TDC)

For the Tunisian double crochet, you will have to yarn over first, then insert the hook for the actual stitch, yarning round the hook and bringing up the loop. Then, you will have to yarn round hook, pulling through the newly-created loop and the initial yarn over, in order to complete the stitch.

If you will do this, you will increase the height of the stitch. In order to create a fabric that is more open, yarn over and work the following two stitches together. For the return pass, the yarn over loops will have to be treated as regular loops.

#9 Tunisian seed stitch (TSS)

The Tunisian seed stitch is known for the ease with which it can be made. Moreover, it can be used to create a nice fabric, with a drape-like effect. In order to begin this particular stitch, for the row forward, you will have to insert the hook at the level of the first chain space.

Then, yarn over and bring up the loop. Insert the hook into the next chain space, yarn over and then withdraw through the loop. Yarn over and pull the work through a number of two loops. The process has to be repeated, until you have only one loop left on the hook.

For the return row, yarn over and withdraw through the loop; then yarn over and withdraw through two loops. Once again, you have to repeat the process, until you only have one loop on the hook. In order to obtain a beautiful pattern, you have to repeat the second row.

#10 Tunisian evelet stitch (TES)

The Tunisian evelet stitch can be used in order to form open spaces (the other alternative is traditional chaining). You can also use this particular type of stitch, in order to create button holes. As you will have the opportunity to see for yourself, the Tunisian evelet stitch will guarantee a different look for the open spaces.

Moreover, you will see that the return horizontal bars actually resemble the Tunisian double-crochet stitches (sideways). In order to make this stitch, all you have to do is make a yarn over for the forward pass. This is valid for each and every stitch that has been skipped. Then, you will have to return using the traditional method.

#11 Tunisian chain lace (TCL)

The Tunisian chain lace is actually a combination of the Tunisian knit stitch with the chain space. The work created with the help of this particular stitch resembles weaved chains. For the first row forward, you will have to skip one chain, then insert the hook in the following chain and bring up one loop. You will have to repeat the process, making sure that all the loops are kept on the hook. For the return row, yarn over and pull the work through the loop.

Then, yarn over and pull the work through two loops. Repeat the process, until you only have one loop on the hook. Another row should be repeated, in order to obtain the desired pattern.

#12 Tunisian queen lace stitch (TQLS)

This Tunisian stitch is similar to the purl stitch, as it requires that the yarn is kept in front of the stitches, before the actual stitch is made. You will have to begin with a traditional foundation row, casting the loops on and off of your hook. The stitch can be made in two ways.

The first requires you to make a yarn over, inserting the hook in the desired stitch; then, you have to repeat the yarn over on and pull up the loop.

The other alternative is to hold the yarn, inserting the hook in the stitch desired and then bring the yarn around the hook. Repeat the yarn over process and then pull up the loop.

The casting off of the stitches can be made in the same way as for the simple Tunisian stitch. You make the yarn over, pulling through the first loop on the hook

Then, you yarn over and pull through two loops. The purpose is to have only one loop remaining on the hook.

#13 Tunisian bubble stitch (TBS)

For the Tunisian bubble stitch, you will have to begin with a traditional foundation row, choosing an odd number of chains. Start by performing a Tunisian simple stitch, then continue with the bubble stitch and finish with another Tunisian simple stitch.

The first step is to make a yarn over, inserting the hook and repeating the yarn over, so as to pull through one loop. Then, yarn over and pull through two loops on the hook. For the second step, yarn over two times, then insert the hook and pull through two loops on the hook (two times as well).

Repeat the process, pull through three loops. Then, cast off the loops, starting with one for the edge and continuing with two, until you only have one loop remaining on the hook. Finish your row with a simple stitch and repeat in order to obtain a beautiful pattern.

#14 Tunisian crossed stitch (TCS)

In order to realize the Tunisian crossed stitch, you will have to begin with an odd number of chain stitches. For the forward pass, for the first row, you will work from right to left. The hook will have to be inserted at the level of the third vertical bar, which means that the first two are going to be skipped. Then, yarn over and bring up the loop (two loops on the hook).

For the next step, the hook will have to be inserted at the level of the second vertical bar (from right to left). Then, yarn over and bring up the loop (three loops on the hook). Repeat the process until you complete the row. For the return pass, you will be working from left to right. Yarn over and bring up the first loop. Then, repeat the process, bringing up two loops at once. The purpose is to have only one remaining loop on the hook. Repeat both passes until you obtain the desired pattern.

#15 Tunisian slip stitch (TSS)

The Tunisian slip stitch is a small crochet stitch and one that is often used for the purpose of practice. You will have to start with a chain that has six stitches, with a slipknot on the hook. The hook will have to be inserted at the level of the first realized chain, leading to the formation of a ring. Then, yarn over and position the hook, so that it faces you.

The hook should be positioned, so that the yarn is used to form the stitch. The hook should be drawn back through the stitch, while the yarn is wrapped on it. Then, it will be drawn once more on the loop on the hook (one single motion required).

Chapter 7 – Tunisian crochet tips and tricks

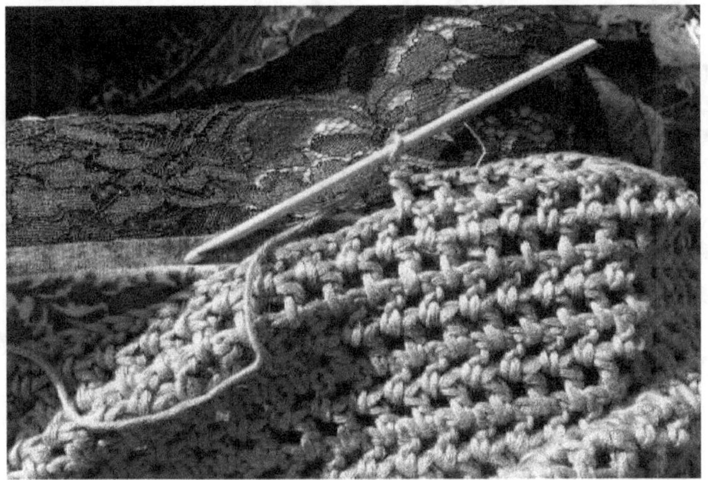

The Tunisian crochet can seem complicated to those who are just beginning to discover it. In order to make this experience easier for you, we have included this chapter, filled with useful tips and tricks. Do not hesitate to read it and apply the advice found in here for an enjoyable crocheting experience.

One of the most important things to keep in mind is that you have to choose a hook that is suitable for your style. As you have seen above, there are different types of hooks available but not all of them are easy to use. Are you going to perform only Tunisian crochet stitches or do you want a hook that will allow you to work in the round as well? Test different types of hooks before you decide on the one that works best for you.

Keep in mind that some types of stitches or patterns require repetitive motions, which can place an excess strain on the hand. In such situations, it is recommended that you choose a hook that has a higher level of flexibility. The double-ended hooks allow you work in the round as well but you can also consider the interchangeable knitting needles. You can prolong the cord, making a shorter or a longer pattern.

If you are going to work in the round, the one thing that you should refrain from doing is twisting the made stitches. In order to avoid such a thing from happening, you will have to pay attention when the chain is joined into the actual round.

The Tunisian crochet experience can be made easier by using a stitch marker. This will allow you to mark the beginning of the round, so that you always remember where you started. There are different types of stitch markers out there but the one that the lock/unlock feature are the best, as they guarantee an easy removal.

Another thing to be on the lookout for is the yarn, as this can easily get tangled. If you are going to work Tunisian crochet in the round, you will require two yarn skeins. In this situation, you will have to keep them separated, as this is the best way to prevent them from getting tangled. A small twist is sufficient, in order for complex tangles to occur, not to mention the nasty knots. Using yarn bowls is the easiest method to prevent such problems. The bowl is useful for preventing the yarn from getting tangled but it also allows you an easy access.

April Showers Shawl

Use a white acrylic yarn with yellow and your Tunisian crochet hook.

Chain 5. Cast these onto your hook. I recommend that you have an extender for you hook if you want to make the shawl larger.

Forward pass single crochet, then return pass with the same. Increase 2 stitches on each side.

Forward pass double crochet, and return pass with the same. Increase by 2 more stitches on each side. Forward pass with single crochet, and return pass with the same.

Continue to do this pattern until you are at the size that you wish your shawl to be, and finish with a nice crocheted border.

If you want to make it more undone, you can add a nice fringe to the bottom of the shawl, and maybe up the sides, too, if you like the way that looks.

Even in the heat of summer, there are still those chilly nights that like to creep up on you. When you are wrapped up in these shawls, you can tell the summer wind to bring on its worst!

You are going to be snug and cozy in these wonderful shawls, and you are going to always have that snug little bit of warmth that you want any time that you need it. Don't' worry about the thunderstorms, or the rain that happens to come up,

you are going to have the perfect solution to anything that can happen, and you are going to look good doing it!

Winter is Coming Shawl

Use brown and white yarn and your Tunisian crochet hook.

Chain 85. Cast these onto your hook. You are probably going to need to have an extender on your hook, or you are going to need to pack them on tightly.

Forward pass single crochet, then return pass with the same. Decrease 2 stitches on each side.

Forward pass double crochet, and return pass with the same. Decrease by 2 more stitches on each side. Forward pass with single crochet, and return pass with the same.

Continue to do this pattern until you are at the size that you wish your shawl to be, and finish with a nice crocheted border.

If you want to make it more undone, you can add a nice fringe to the bottom of the shawl, and maybe up the sides, too, if you like the way that looks.

Turning Leaves Shawl

Use a green and brown yarn and the Tunisian crochet hook.

Chain 12. Cast these onto your Tunisian crochet hook, and single crochet for your forward and return passes all the way across the rows.

You are going to increase steadily with each row, so you are going to have to pay attention to your stitches as well as your tension. This is a shawl that has a wide base, but you are going to continue to work until the top of it is much wider.

This is a shawl that is up to you to make it the size that you want it to be. Continue to increase with each side by 2 stitches for each row, and when you are done with the main body of the shawl, you can switch to your other crochet hook and the brown yarn.

Crochet a brown border around the edge of the shawl, and use your yarn needle to make the stem of the leaf. Have fun and put in the details that you want, and you can make it as leaf like as you want.

You can also use a green for the border, but make sure that this is a different green than the one that you were using, so you can still see the details that you put on.

Midsummer Night Shawl

Use a black light weight yarn and your Tunisian crochet hook.

Chain 145. Cast these onto your Tunisian crochet hook, and begin your first forward pass.

Single crochet in each stitch from the hook, then for your return pass, single crochet in one, skip one chain 1, and single crochet in the next stitch. Chain 1, skip the next stitch, and single crochet in the next stitch.

Skip 1, chain 1, and single crochet in the next stitch. Repeat this for your entire return pass, then again for the forward pass.

This pattern isn't going to have any increases or decreases, so keep your tension even and your count spot on. Skip one, chain one, crochet in the next one. You are making a checkered pattern that is going to be made of holes and openings, but not large holes or openings.

Keep working until you are happy with the size of the shawl, then cast off the stitches. Single crochet around the entire border, then chain 1 and turn, single crochet in the first stitch from the hook.

Chain 1 and skip 1, then single crochet in the next stitch. Repeat this your entire way around the shawl, and when you reach the end, tie off securely.

Misty Breeze Shawl

Use a sport weight yarn in a light green color, and your Tunisian crochet hook.

Chain 12. Cast on to your Tunisian crochet hook. Forward pass single crochet across the row, then return pass single crochet across the row.

Repeat this until you have completed 8 rows. Tie off.

Chain 18. Cast on to your Tunisian crochet hook, then forward pass double crochet across the row. Return pass the same way, and keep going until you have reached 8 rows. Tie off.

Do this once more with 24 stitches to begin with, and single crochet, then again with 32 stitches, and double crochet. Then 36 stitches, and single crochet, and 45 stitches, double crochet.

When you have all of your patterns done, lay out the panels, and sew up the ends. You want to lay them so that they are centered, and you can see the increases without having to actually put in any of the increases.

When you have all of the panels sewn together, use your crochet hook to make a nice border around the edge of the shawl. You may want to make a few rows for the border so it has more of a complete look.

Tie off when you are finished.

If you are planning on using the double-ended crochet hook, keep in mind that the stitches are required to be worked in groups. This is because the hook lacks the necessary flexibility for an entire round. So, when you move from one group to the other, it is a good idea that you leave a couple of stitches unworked (at the end of each group). In this way, you will obtain a seamless appearance.

In the situation that you have problems with curling, there are several actions you can take. First and foremost, you have the process known as blocking. As it was mentioned above, blocking is one of the easiest steps that you can take, in order to give your work the desired form. You can steam it with the help of the iron or even wet it, waiting for the work to dry and achieve the intended form. Easy and fast, that is what blocking is all about.

Another way to prevent excessive curling is by using a bigger hook, as this will reduce how much tension there is in your work. The more you reduce this tension, the more reduced the chance for curling is going to be. If you cannot find a hook of a larger size, you can modify the foundation chain.

 In order to do this, the foundation chain has to be turned and the loops pulled through the back ridge of each individual chain. You can find the back ridge in the background of two chain loops (characteristic V shape). Apart from preventing curling, this process also guarantees a clean and organized finish of your work (at the edge).

In order to take the curl out of the Tunisian crochet, you can also consider using other types of stitches for the beginning rows. For example, the purl stitch guarantees the least amount of curling, in comparison to other types of Tunisian stitches. You can even attempt to perform the first rows using this particular stitch, before starting with the actual pattern you want to create.

The Tunisian crochet is perfect for working with multiple yarn colors. The good news is that the colors can be changed in the middle of the row, so that you are able to create intricate patterns. It is also worth mentioning that the yarn does not have to be cut when you are switching colors; instead, you can carry one color along the edge of the respective row, until you use it for the next row. Basically, you do not have to worry weaving, which is great.

The yarn choice is also important, especially if you want your project to turn out as desired. When shopping for yarn, it is a good idea to read the label, so that you obtain all the necessary information. You can find out details on the fabric from which the yarn is made and also decide on the fabric, according to the project for which you require it.

For example, wool is recommended for outdoor wear, such as scarves or hats. On the other hand, cotton and bamboo are especially recommended for kids.

These are some of the tips and tricks that can improve your Tunisian crochet experience. Do not hesitate to use them and enjoy your new hobby. Without doubt, it will contribute to the appearance of beautiful projects, whether we are talking about scarves, hats, shawls, baby blankets or pillow cases.

Chapter 8 – Tunisian Crochet Projects

You don't have to be in the mountains to know that springtime is one of the wettest and coldest times of the year. You can wrap up in any of these shawls and you are going to be warm and snug no matter what is coming your way!

When you have these shawls, you are going to have instant access to any number of warmth that you could ever want. You are going to be ready to face the rain and the late winter snow, and you are going to stave off those chilly winds that are going to cut through any of the clothes that you have on.

With these shawls, you are going to be ready for anything, and you aren't going to have to worry about winter, or spring, or any of the elements that come up again!

With your shawl and a cup of coffee, you are set!

Spring Rain Shawl

Use a light blue sport weight yarn and your Tunisian crochet hook.

Chain 120. Cast on with your Tunisian crochet hook. If you need more room, extenders can be purchased at a craft store, or you can work in with strips as you did with the last crochet hook.

Forward pass with double crochet, then switch to single crochet for your return pass. Repeat this with another forward pass and double crochet, then skip the first 3 stitches when you do the return pass and single crochet. Stop working when you are 3 stitches away from the end.

Forward pass and double crochet in each stitch on the next row, then return pass skipping the first 2 stitches on the hook. Stop before you reach the last 2 stitches on the other end.

Forward pass with double crochet, and skip the first 2 when you make your return pass and single crochet.

You can see with this pattern that you are decreasing steadily the entire way down the rows until you reach the point of only having a few stitches left. You don't want it to be a single stitch point, so you should stop when you have about 5 or 6 stitches left.

When you are at the point at the bottom of your shawl, cast off and tie off your lose end. Use your Tunisian crochet hook, or any crochet hook that you prefer to crochet a finishing border around the edge of the shawl.

Tie off and you are ready to wear!

Dances in the Rain Shawl

Use a Tunisian crochet hook and an acrylic yarn in the color of your choice.

Chain 24. Cast these onto your hook, and single crochet forward pass along the row. Return pass with double crochet, then return pass with triple crochet.

Forward pass once more with single crochet, then return pass with double crochet, then forward pass with triple crochet. You can see what this pattern is, and continue to do it until your strip is as long as you want your shawl to be wide.

Tie off and repeat this, starting with triple crochet as the forward pass, double crochet as the return pass, then single crochet as the forward pass.

Repeat this for 3 more panels, then use your crochet hook to sew them all together, and crochet a nice border.

Fall nights are the chilliest ones that are around. When you are wrapped up in your shawl, you are warm and cozy no matter what the world outside is doing. So what are you waiting for?

There is a whole new world of shawls out there that are just waiting for you to make them up and wrap around you for the chilly nights that are to come! You are going to fall in love with the warmth, as well as the looks of these cozy shawls.

Don't fear the chilly nights anymore, you now have the key to anything warmth you will ever need!

Fireside Nights Shawl

Use a brown and red yarn and your Tunisian crochet hook.

Chain 5. Cast these onto your hook. Single crochet a thin strip that is 5 stitches long and about 5 feet long.

Forward pass single crochet, then return pass with the same. This is going to be a shawl that alternates single and double, the first strip being single and the second being double.

For the second panel, you are going to use double crochet, but you are going to maintain the pattern of 5 stitches on your hook and 5 feet long. Remember that you are going to alternate colors as well as texture.

Make the single crochet panels brown, and the double crochet panels red. When you have enough to make the shawl the size that you want it to be, tie off and sew all of them together.

Add on a border of the brown first, then the red, alternating for 4 rows and using single crochet. Tie off and you are ready to wrap up in a bundle of warmth!

Shawls are the one thing that we all wish that we had on a cold winter night. Now, you can have one for every night of the week, because you can mix and match to make them your own.

These are all shawls that are meant to be warm. Make one for you or your daughter, or your mother or your grandmother. Each and every one of you is going to fall in love with the warmth that these provide, and the wonderful memories that they build up when you are making them.

You can have fun together, all wrapped up in your shawls that you made yourself. Who needs to go to the store or buy into the ideas that they are trying to sell you on the television? When you are able to make your own shawls, you can make the how you want them when you want them.

There is no need to stick to the rules or to be afraid to change it up to suit your needs, when you are making them yourself, you are able to make them how you want. It is like the perfect freedom to have the only shawl that is like that in the whole world, and it is a piece of beauty.

I know you are going to love these wonderful winter shawls, and they are going to bring tons of memories for you and anyone that you make them for.

Snowman Shawl

Use a white yarn with black and orange to garnish and your Tunisian crochet hook.

Chain 200. Make sure that you use your extender for this one, you are going to need it. Cast on these stitches onto your hook, and forward pass your single crochet.

Decreases by 2 on each side, and single crochet your return pass. Forward pass once more with your single crochet, then return pass again, with both passes, you need to be decreasing by 2.

Continue to forward pass and return pass with your decreases and single crochet, until you reach a nice point at the bottom. One that is 5 or 6 stitches across.

Use the black to single crochet a border around the edge of the entire shawl, and sue your yarn needle to stitch in eyes and a nose with the orange and black.

Tie off securely, and you are ready to show off your wonderful new frosty the snowman shawl!

Along the Lane Shawl

Use a white yarn in acrylic or sport weight and a Tunisian crochet hook.

Chain 7 and cast on to your Tunisian crochet hook. This entire pattern is worked in double crochet.

Increase by 2 stitches on both sides, and work a single double crochet row per increase. Forward pass and return pass, making certain that your tension is even and that you aren't pulling in on the yarn in any way.

When you have reached the size that you want your shawl to be, crochet a border around the edge of the entire shawl.

This is also a pretty shawl to be worked with blue incorporated as the border, or if you decide to use blue as the body of the shawl.

Have fun and decide what color you like best, and you are set!

Insider's tip: It can be difficult to work with Tunisian crochet when you use two strands of yarn held together, so it is recommended that you avoid doing this when you are working in Tunisian crochet.

If you want to make a multi-colored shawl in the body of the shawl, you should use your yarn needle to add in features, or you could make panels of different colors then sew those together. Obviously, the easiest way to do this is to use a multi-colored yarn from the beginning of the pattern, or to plan on keeping the shawl as one color for the body, then adding in a different color for the border or for finer details like that.

Christmas Lights Shawl

Use a green acrylic yarn and your Tunisian crochet hook.

Christmas lights are all different colors, so you can use any color that you want, or you can add in a multi-colored yarn when you are finishing the project, we went for the feel of an actual Christmas tree with this one so we used the green for the main color.

Start by chaining 200. Cast on with an extender on the end of your hook, and forward pass triple crochet. Return pass triple crochet as well, decreases by 2 stitches on each side.

Continue to use triple crochet on each row, and decrease by 2 stitches on each side as you work your way down the shawl. You can stop at any time that you feel the shawl is big enough, but we recommend that you continue to work down until you have reached a fine point at the end of the shawl.

With this shawl, we went into a much finer point than we did with the other shawl patterns, and this is because Christmas trees are brought to an actual point at the top of them.

When you are ready, you can use the multi-colored yarn of your choice for the border. This is going to be the light effect on your shawl, so go with a color that you are happy with, and one that you are going to be proud to wear. You can use this as just the border, or you can use it as an intertwine for your entire shawl.

However you decide to do it, have fun and make your shawl exactly as you want it to be!

It might be summer, it might be winter, or it might be a season in between the two, you are still feeling chilly and you would love to have that little bit of warmth to wrap yourself up in.

Or perhaps you know that Christmas is coming, and you want to be able to give that perfect gift to all of the little girls and girlfriends that you have, but you don't know what that would be, until you tried on one of these wonderful shawls.

When the Weather Outside is Frightful Shawl

Use the color of your choice in acrylic and your Tunisian crochet hook.

Start by chaining 20, and cast this onto your Tunisian crochet hook. Work your first panel with single crochet only as you forward pass and return pass, making sure that your tension is a constant even, and that you aren't pulling in.

You want this to be about 18 inches long, then tie it off.

Chain 20 for your next panel. Use double crochet, and forward and return pass the same as you did in the first panel. Keep your tension even and don't pull in on it when you are in the middle. This is a common mistake that a lot of first time crochet artists make.

Stop when your panel is 24 inches long. Then work the next panel as 20 inches to begin with and triple crochet. You are going to work the forward and return passes as always, with even tension and paying attention to make sure that you don't pull in on the center of the pattern.

When you reach 30 inches, tie it off, and make a fourth panel that is 20 stiches, and single crochet. Stop with this one when you reach 36 inches, and the next when you reach 42. Finally, finish the last panel with triple crochet and an even 50 inches.

Lay out your panels on the table in descending order, and sew up the ends so they are together as one piece, use your crochet hook and crochet a border on the edge, evening it all up so you don't have the large blocks hanging off the end.

You are going to need to do more than one row of border to ensure that it all looks even. Tie off and you are ready to strut your stuff!

Wrapped in Warmth Shawl

Use a brown or an orange in acrylic and your Tunisian crochet hook.

Chain 175. Use an extension on your hook, and cast all of these stitches onto your hook. Single crochet your forward pass and double crochet your return pass.

You are going to work a single crochet forward pass and a double crochet return pass for each of the rows before you decrease. When you do decrease, you are going to decrease by 3 stitches on each side of the shawl.

Then you need to remember to do the 2 rows of double crochet, and decrease once more. Continue to keep your tension even, it is a tendency to pull the yarn tight when you are decreasing to make the decrease more obvious, but I can assure you that it is all going to look right when you reach the bottom of the shawl.

Continue to work until you are at the fine point at the bottom of the shawl. You can stop when you have a nice rounded edge, or you can continue to work until you have a fine point at the bottom of the shawl.

No matter what you decide, when you are at the bottom of the shawl, tie it off and crochet a border around the edge of the entire shawl. Work a couple of rows for the border so you can keep it all looking deliberate and even, and you are set!

Because You Need a Hug Shawl

Use a soft yarn in the color of your choice and your Tunisian crochet hook.

Take note that it can be more difficult to work with a soft yarn, so try to avoid the ones that are very bulky or the ones that are easily snagged on items that are around your home.

As soon as you have settled on a yarn, you are ready to begin. Chain 120. Work a simple single crochet forward pass, then return pass with another single crochet. You are going to continue to work with single crochet, but you need to watch to make sure that your tension is even and that you don't miss any stitches on your way down.

Decrease by a single stitch on each side of the shawl for each row that you are working, and you are going to see a steady decrease on your way down. When you are at the bottom of the shawl, tie it off and work in the loose end.

You have to be careful with soft yarn as it tends to stay bulky at the bottom of the project. Work in the ends, and crochet a nice border around the edge of the shawl, and you are ready to go!

I hope that you enjoyed each of these shawls, and it is important to remember that each and every project takes practice. Work at it until you get it, and you are going to become a master. The more you work, the easier it is going to become.

Have fun and explore what you can do, and you are going to be amazed at the things that you can come up with!

Chapter 9 – Fun and Fancy Projects

There is always a lot of fun in being able to design your own things. This is true no matter what you want to make. Whether it be something that you keep in your house, or something that you wear, the ability to design something all on your own is a major part of the fun.

Western Dog Collar

Measure the length of your dog's collar. Make a foundation chain that is 2 inches wide and Tunisian crochet a strip that is as long as your dog's collar, plus 3 inches.

Using the same color, repeat these steps, until you have 2 strips. Then, using a different color, make a third strip.

Tie them all off securely, then, using a yarn needle, sew the base of them together. Once they are all joined, braid the strips together. Lay them flat so they are braiding in a flat strip, and sew a bit in the middle so they are secured at each point they cross.

Once you have reached three fourths of the way up, sew in a ring to slip the braid through when you are finished. Continue to braid up the entire piece, then sew the end together securely.

Tie it off, and you are ready to go! Slip it around your dog's neck and be ready to walk the streets in style!

Celebrity Clutch

This is a smaller project, so you will want to use a lighter weight yarn. There are all kinds of novelty yarns you can purchase at any crafting store, but there is also the old standby of sport weight yarn if you choose to go with a slightly easier material to work with.

Using sport weight yarn (or whatever yarn you choose to work with) make a foundation chain that is 5 inches wide. Continue with your Tunisian crochet until it is 7 inches long as well. Fold in half and set aside.

Now, using regular crochet, make a strip that is 5 inches wide but only 3 inches long. This is then sewn inside the first flap. Make sure that you line up the bottom with the edges of the clutch and sew them on evenly.

Now, make another rectangle, only make this one 5 inches wide by 4 inches long. Sew this one in the other side, then, using a yarn needle, sew in compartments to keep your cards.

Secure the closure with a big button, and you are ready to sport your clutch anywhere that you go! If you want to make it that much more classy, then slip stitch a little loop to make a handle for you to hang onto.

Spider Web Blanket

This is a pattern that is a little harder than the other ones we have been looking at so far. You may be familiar with chain 1 and skipping one, or chaining 2 and skipping 2, but did you know that you can do the same thing with Tunisian crochet?

This is the same, simple, granny square pattern that we have been doing, only this time you are going to go through your first row, then you are going to do the same chain 1 skip 1 pattern.

It works the same way as regular crochet, you just have to keep an eye on where you are in the project. Follow this pattern carefully, and you will see that it works the same way.

If you are not getting the drape that you would like to see, increase the stitches in between, so you are chaining 2 or 3 and skipping as many.

Once you have enough squares, sew them together as you would a regular granny square blanket. When it is all finished, add plenty of fringe to the sides. This is a cute Halloween throw, make the squares out of black or orange, and contrast them with the other color.

A pure white blanket is beautiful as well.

Chapter 10 – Projects for Your House

What could be better than making things that you can also use around the house? There are so many little trinkets that you have to indulge in, how can you let those things slip by and not have to embellish them with things that are also homemade.

These are patterns that you can make to use around your house. They are all easy and exotic, making them the perfect addition to your Tunisian collection. Your guests will be amazed at how beautiful your pieces are, and what you can make with your imagination.

You don't have to tell them how easy it really is to do this, just let them wonder at how you are able to put together such lovely pieces in so many ways. There are few things more satisfying than being able to look around your house and see things that you made yourself.

Runway Rug

Make a foundation chain that is 2 inches wide, then begin your long strip of Tunisian crochet. Do this until you have a length of chain that is about 20 feet long.

This will take some time, but be patient, you need to make sure that it is long enough for you to wrap around several times, or else it won't lie properly. Once you have your length, make sure you tie it off completely, then you are ready to begin wrapping.

Wrap it around itself several times, all the while securing it with yarn through a yarn needle. It will make it lie a lot flatter if you do this while you go along. Once you have the whole rug assembled, steam it.

Lay the whole thing on your ironing board, and let the steam run over it until it is soft and pliable. Then, attach rubber rug stoppers on the bottom of the rug so it doesn't slide about as you use it.

Beautiful Bath Mat

Using cotton, make a foundation chain that is 2 feet wide. Then, make a row of Tunisian crochet that then measures 3 feet long by 2 feet wide. Once this is completed, tie it off and set it aside.

When that is done, make another rectangle the same way, only this time make it out of an acrylic and cotton blend. You can do this by holding the two pieces together.

Once you have your second rectangle, lay that one on top of the first and sew them together. Then, using your yarn needle, sew through the middle of the rug in various places so they hold together.

When you have it all secured, flip the rug over so the blended side is on top, and the cotton side is on the bottom. Add a nice fringe to the sides of the rug, and rug stoppers to the bottom.

Once it is all secure, you are ready to use it!

Insider's tip: If you want it to hold the fringe better, twist them together and make miniature ropes off of the end of the bath mat. This will also give the project a more nautical feel.

Placemats

You don't have to limit yourself to yarn fiber when you are doing this kind of crochet any more than if you were doing regular crochet. Feel free to explore. While this is a project that can be made out of any material, we recommend using hemp or a hemp blend.

This is a really simple design, but it adds great beauty to your table. Make a foundation chain that is 15 inches wide, then, using every other row for a pattern, Tunisian crochet the first row, then double crochet the second.

Make sure you are chaining 2 at the end of every row, and that you turn when you are doing the double crochet. Otherwise, don't worry about turning your project.

Once you have it the size that you want it, tie it off and make as many as you need for the guests that you have.

Dish Soap Skirt

Who doesn't like to dress up their dish soap? This fun and flirty project makes your soap fashionable and fun while you do the dishes.

Make a small foundation chain, one that is the length of the bottom of your bottle of dish detergent. Decrease the same as you would with regular crochet, and work your way up the bottle in a slow triangle.

When you reach the top, tie it off, then cut 4 pieces of yarn to attach to the top and bottom, then tie it onto your bottle of soap like an apron. This is sure to spruce up any bottle and add a bit of charm to any kitchen sink!

There are always those projects that never seem to fit in any category. That's ok though, everyone needs their misfits in society. That is exactly what these projects are, but they are sure to fit into your day quite nicely!

Table Runner

You don't need to have an occasion to have a table runner, these charming little pieces brighten up any living room or dining room table. This one is going to have a bit of a foreign flair to it with your Tunisian crochet.

Start with a foundation chain of 3, and slowly increase on each side until your runner measures 5 inches across. If you are having a difficult time with this in Tunisian crochet, simply use single crochet.

Once you reach the wide part, use Tunisian crochet until you are at the other end. Go back to your standard of single crochet to finish it off, and you are set!

Doily

Keep an open pattern with this one, and make sure you use a lighter weight yarn. This is something that does take practice, but you will get it if you are consistent and work with what you have.

This is a simple square, make your foundation chain as long as you want it, then Tunisian crochet all the way across until you have a nice square. This is really open, so you need to chain 4 in between all of your stitches.

When you reach the end, add lots of fringe for that classy look. There are few things more charming than a doily with something nice and neat on it. Make sure your shelves aren't bare with these charming little doilies all over the top of them.

Flags

You can make these singular, or you can make them and sew them together in a chain and make them a banner. Either way they're the perfect addition to any wall or door.

Start at the widest point, and make a foundation chain about 5 inches wide. Now, Tunisian crochet as we showed you, only decrease as you go down the chain.

Then, make sure you come to a point at the bottom and tie it off when you get there.

Sew the flags together tip to tip until you have a nice string of triangles, and you are set to hang it anywhere in your home for all to see!

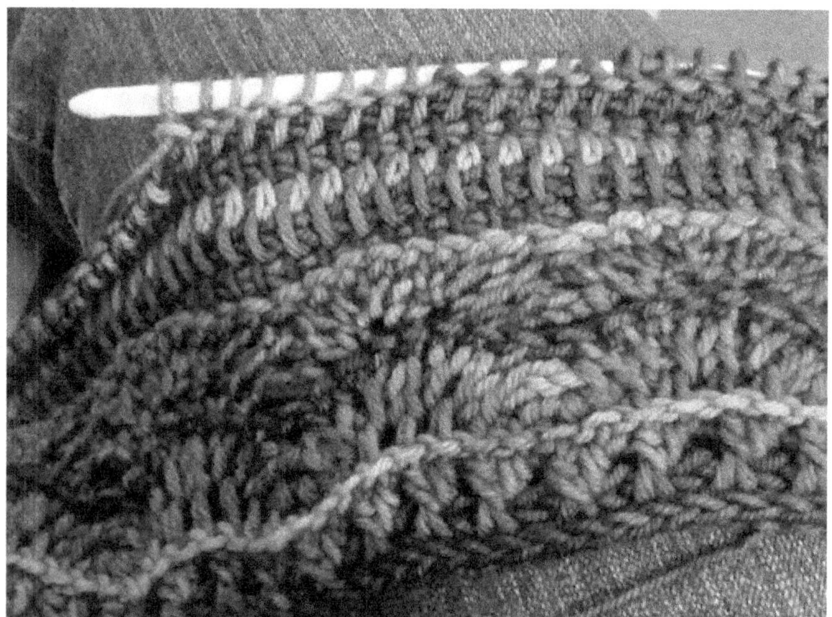

Plushy Throw

Use a large hook and baby soft yarn for this one. It comes in many different colors, you just have to get it at the crafting store.

This is a project that is worked as one large square. It is made as you would make an afghan throw in knitting. Chain 290 for your foundation chain, and go up from there.

If you want to make it a little more varied, you can add in regular crochet at random places, just make sure that you are consistent with it, and that you are chaining extra at the beginning every time you chain a regular crochet.

What better way to wrap up this book than with these charming little projects. By the time you have completed these, you have finished all of the 20 projects that we had in here for you, but you are going to need to still work on your skills to make sure you have them all down well.

Take your time and work at these nicely, when you feel that you have them down, then you can move on in your skill.

Curtains

This is a simple pattern for an elaborate project. You will be amazed at how easy it is to make the perfect custom curtains for any room, and all you have to do is a single stitch.

Measure how long your current curtains are when they are completely flat. Then, you make a foundation chain that long. When you are working your way down, make sure that you add on an extra 5 inches to the rectangle.

Then, fold that flap over, and in half, and sew it in place. Now you should have a tube to feed the rod through.

Feed the rod through the tube and make sure it is all gathered. That's it! They are ready to hang.

Cell Bag

For those of us who have smart phones that we want to dress smart. Use a multi-colored yarn with this one, and you will only have to use a single stitch for a beautiful pattern!

Measure your smart phone. For the iPhones, make a foundation chain that is 4 inches wide, then Tunisian crochet 5 inches high. Tie it off, then repeat this process with a second one.

Once they are both complete, sew them together with wide pieces of string, creating a fringe the whole way up the side of the case.

Insider's tip: If you want more security, sew the pieces together before you add on the fringe. It will look the same, but it will also add more security so you don't accidentally lose your phone out of the side.

Wrist Bands and Bracelets

For these, make the same kind of strip that you did for the dog collar, only make them a lot shorter. If you are going to braid them you need only use a couple of pieces and twist them together.

It can be difficult to braid a bracelet that is so thick, so for these Tunisian crocheted strips, simply sew them together on the side, and leave extra string at the end so you can tie them together for wear.

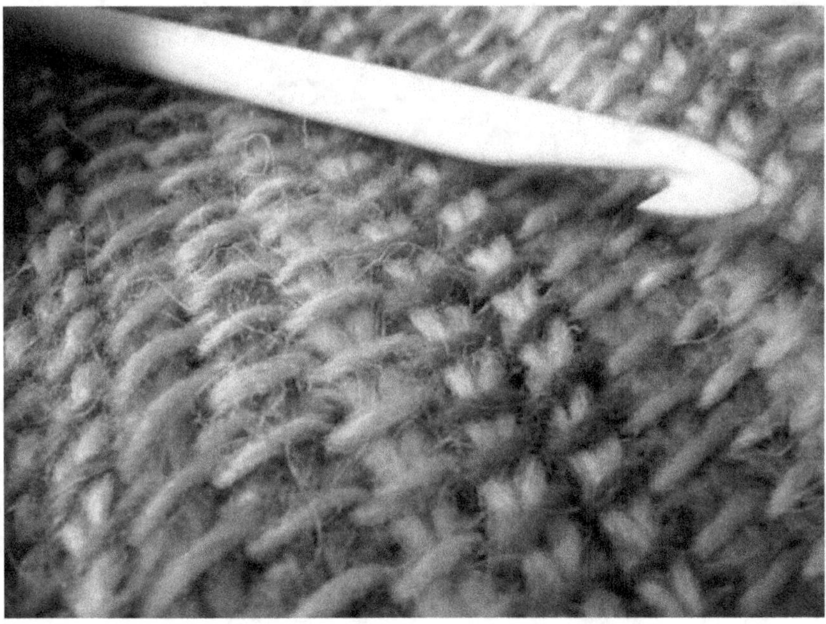

Headbands

These are beautiful accessories to wear any time of the year, but keep in mind that they do get hot, so you don't want to make them out of anything too heavy. Sport weight or cotton is a good choice.

Make a foundation chain that is 4 inches wide, then Tunisian crochet a long strip, about 6 inches in length total. Leave strings on the end to tie it together, and wear it either over your ears or across your forehead.

This is a fun and flirty design for any length of hair, and even men can wear it. Make one in every color, and some in multi-color to make sure you have one for every occasion!

Conclusion

There you have it, you have now joined in the wonderful and magical world of Tunisian crochet. It is as though you are able to travel to another country every time you get into your crafting bag.

These projects are all just the beginning, once you are able to get on to the next level, there is no stopping you or what you can make. This is an incredible opportunity to make everything you want out of yarn in a style that is out of the ordinary.

Make things for your friends and family, and never have to worry about another gift giving event again. This is your opportunity to make the most elaborate and stunning projects out of very little materials.

Don't get discouraged if it takes you a while to get the hang of things. This is a craft that takes practice, but it is one that is also easy to pick up on once you got it. There is no end to the ways you can express yourself.

Don't rush things, and make sure you have your tension even and firm throughout. This is the best way to make sure it is going to come out even and natural.

Don't worry if you can't get it at first. No one does. This is a skill that comes with time and practice, but I know that you will get it if you stick with it and don't give up!